Obstetric and Gynecologic Hospitalists and Laborists

Editors

BRIGID McCUE
JENNIFER A. TESSMER-TUCK

OBSTETRICS AND GYNECOLOGY CLINICS OF NORTH AMERICA

www.obgyn.theclinics.com

Consulting Editor
WILLIAM F. RAYBURN

September 2015 • Volume 42 • Number 3

ELSEVIER

1600 John F. Kennedy Boulevard • Suite 1800 • Philadelphia, Pennsylvania, 19103-2899

http://www.theclinics.com

OBSTETRICS AND GYNECOLOGY CLINICS OF NORTH AMERICA Volume 42, Number 3
September 2015 ISSN 0889-8545, ISBN-13: 978-0-323-39575-5

Editor: Kerry Holland
Developmental Editor: Kristen Helm

Obstetrics and Gynecology Clinics (ISSN 0889-8545) is published quarterly by Elsevier Inc., 360 Park Avenue South, New York, NY 10010-1710. Months of issue are March, June, September, and December. Periodicals postage paid at New York, NY, and additional mailing offices. Subscription price per year is $310.00 (US individuals), $545.00 (US institutions), $155.00 (US students), $370.00 (Canadian individuals), $688.00 (Canadian institutions), $225.00 (Canadian students), $450.00 (international individuals), $688.00 (international institutions), and $225.00 (international students). To receive student/resident rate, orders must be accompanied by name of affiliated institution, date of term, and the signature of program/residency coordinator on institution letterhead. Orders will be billed at individual rate until proof of status is received. Foreign air speed delivery is included in all *Clinics* subscription prices. All prices are subject to change without notice. POSTMASTER: Send address changes to *Obstetrics and Gynecology Clinics*, Elsevier Health Sciences Division, Subscription Customer Service, 3251 Riverport Lane, Maryland Heights, MO 63043. **Customer Service: Telephone: 1-800-654-2452 (U.S. and Canada); 314-447-8871 (outside U.S. and Canada). Fax: 314-447-8029. E-mail: journalscustomerservice-usa@elsevier.com (for print support); journalsonlinesupport-usa@elsevier. com (for online support).**

Reprints. For copies of 100 or more of articles in this publication, please contact the Commercial Reprints Department, Elsevier Inc., 360 Park Avenue South, New York, New York 10010-1710. Tel.: 212-633-3874; Fax: 212-633-3820; E-mail: reprints@elsevier.com.

Obstetrics and Gynecology Clinics of North America is also published in Spanish by McGraw-Hill Interamericana Editores S.A., P.O. Box 5-237, 06500, Mexico; in Portuguese by Reichmann and Affonso Editores, Rio de Janeiro, Brazil; and in Greek by Paschalidis Medical Publications, Athens, Greece.

Obstetrics and Gynecology Clinics of North America is covered in MEDLINE/PubMed (Index Medicus), Excerpta Medica, Current Concepts/Clinical Medicine, Science Citation Index, BIOSIS, CINAHL, and ISI/BIOMED.

Contributors

CONSULTING EDITOR

WILLIAM F. RAYBURN, MD, MBA
Associate Dean, Continuing Medical Education and Professional Development, Distinguished Professor and Emeritus Chair, Obstetrics and Gynecology, University of New Mexico School of Medicine, Albuquerque, New Mexico

EDITORS

BRIGID MCCUE, MD, PhD
Chief, Department of Obstetrics, Gynecology, and Midwifery, Beth Israel Deaconess Hospital–Plymouth, Plymouth, Massachusetts

JENNIFER A. TESSMER-TUCK, MD
Clinical Program Director, Women and Children's Services, Medical Director, North Memorial Laborist Associates, Department of Obstetrics and Gynecology, North Memorial Health Care, Robbinsdale, Minnesota

AUTHORS

ROBERT M. ABRAMS, MD
Associate Professor, Division of Maternal Fetal Medicine, Department of Obstetrics and Gynecology, Southern Illinois University School of Medicine, Springfield, Illinois

STEVEN L. CLARK, MD
Professor, Maternal Fetal Medicine, Department of Obstetrics and Gynecology, Baylor College of Medicine, Houston, Texas

THOMAS J. GARITE, MD
Professor Emeritus, University of California, Irvine, Orange, California; Director of Research and Education, Obstetrics MedNax/Pediatrix Medical Group; Chief Medical Officer, Perigen Inc, Sunrise, Florida

ERIC E. HOWELL, MD
Associate Professor of Medicine, Division of Hospital Medicine, Department of Medicine, Johns Hopkins Bayview Medical Center, Johns Hopkins University School of Medicine, Baltimore, Maryland

BRIAN K. IRIYE, MD
Managing Partner, High Risk Pregnancy Center; Chair, Association for Maternal Fetal Medicine Management, Las Vegas, Nevada

FLORA KISUULE, MD, MPH
Assistant Professor of Medicine, Division of Hospital Medicine, Department of Medicine, Johns Hopkins Bayview Medical Center, Johns Hopkins University School of Medicine, Baltimore, Maryland

LISA LEVINE, MD, MSCE
Department of Obstetrics and Gynecology, Perelman School of Medicine, University of Pennsylvania, Philadelphia, Pennsylvania

BRIGID MCCUE, MD, PhD
Chief, Department of Obstetrics, Gynecology, and Midwifery, Beth Israel Deaconess Hospital–Plymouth, Plymouth, Massachusetts

JORDAN MESSLER, MD, SFHM
Incompass Health, Morton Plant Hospital, Clearwater, Florida

BRIAN MONKS, MD
Medical Director of Practice Development, Ob Hospitalist Group, Ob Hospitalist, North Austin Medical Center, Austin, Texas

ROB OLSON, MD
Founding President, Society of OB/GYN Hospitalists, Peace Health St. Joseph Medical Center, Editor, ObGynHospitalist.com, Bellingham, Washington

WILLIAM F. RAYBURN, MD, MBA
Associate Dean, Continuing Medical Education and Professional Development, Distinguished Professor and Emeritus Chair, Obstetrics and Gynecology, University of New Mexico School of Medicine, Albuquerque, New Mexico

MARK SIMON, MD, MMM
Vice President of Medical Affairs, Ob Hospitalist Group, Inc, Mauldin, South Carolina

SINDHU K. SRINIVAS, MD, MSCE
Assistant Professor, Department of Obstetrics and Gynecology, Perelman School of Medicine, University of Pennsylvania, Philadelphia, Pennsylvania

TOBEY A. STEVENS, MD
Assistant Professor, Department of Obstetrics and Gynecology, OB/GYN Hospitalist, Baylor College of Medicine, Houston, Texas

LAURIE S. SWAIM, MD
Associate Professor, Director, Division of Gynecologic and Obstetric Specialists, Department of Obstetrics and Gynecology, Baylor College of Medicine, Houston, Texas

CHRISTOPHER SWAIN, MD, FACOG
Chief Medical Officer and Founder, Ob Hospitalist Group, Inc, Mauldin, South Carolina

JENNIFER A. TESSMER-TUCK, MD
Clinical Program Director, Women and Children's Services, Medical Director, North Memorial Laborist Associates, Department of Obstetrics and Gynecology, North Memorial Health Care, Robbinsdale, Minnesota

LARRY VELTMAN, MD, CPHRM, FACOG
Risk Management and Perinatal Safety Consultant, Portland, Oregon

ANTHONY M. VINTZILEOS, MD
Chairman, Department of Obstetrics and Gynecology, Winthrop University Hospital, Mineola, New York; Professor of Obstetrics, Gynecology and Reproductive Medicine, Stony Brook University School of Medicine, New York, New York

LOUIS WEINSTEIN, MD
Past Bowers Professor and Chair, Department of Obstetrics and Gynecology, Thomas Jefferson University, Philadelphia, Pennsylvania

WINTHROP F. WHITCOMB, MD, MHM
Remedy Partners, Darien, Connecticut

Contents

The laborist model offers the best approach to standardize care and improve patient safety on the labor unit, improve physician well-being, and decrease physician dissatisfaction/burnout. The concept of the laborist was based on the hospitalist model. The laborist is free of the stresses of a private practice, works a constant and controllable schedule, and can have work shift limitations, thereby eliminating the issue of fatigue and impairment, and improving patient safety while decreasing the potential for adverse outcomes that may result in a liability action. This is what is being demanded both by patients and generation Y physicians.

Hospitalists work in 90% of US hospitals with over 200 beds. With over 48,000 practicing hospitalists nationwide, the field of hospital medicine has grown rapidly in its 20 years of existence. Obstetrics and gynecology (OBGYN) hospitalists are uncovering similar drivers for their growth. Obstetricians cannot be in both the hospital and the office at the same time, they face an increased acuity of hospitalized patients demanding a full time presence, and hospitals are searching for physicians aligned with their goals. OBGYN hospitalists are at a similar point today at which hospital medicine was in the late 1990s.

The forces promoting the hospitalist model arose from the need for high-value care; therefore, improving quality and cost has been part of the hospitalist formula for success. The factors driving the rapid growth of generalist and subspecialty hospitalists include nationally mandated quality and safety measures, increasing age and complexity of the hospitalized patient, reduced residency duty hours, increased economic pressures to contain costs and reduce length of stay, and also primary care physicians, and specialists, relinquishing hospital privileges to focus on outpatient practices. Hospitalists are playing key roles in patient safety and quality as either leaders or practitioners in the field.

decision to delivery. Further study is needed on maternal and neonatal outcomes to corroborate earlier observations, and to closely examine the type of obstetric hospitalist model being observed to aid in planning the ideal deployment of providers in this workforce of the future.

Staffing models are critical aspects of care delivery. Provider staffing on the labor and delivery unit has recently received heightened attention. Based on the general medicine hospitalist model, the obstetrics and gynecology hospitalist or laborist model of obstetric care was introduced more than a decade ago as a plausible model-of-care delivery to improve provider satisfaction with the goal of also improving safety and outcomes through continuous coverage by providers whose sole focus was on the labor and delivery unit without other competing clinical duties. It is plausible that this model of provider staffing and care delivery will increase safety.

Sleep deprivation occurs when inadequate sleep leads to decreased performance, inadequate alertness, and deterioration in health. It is incompletely understood why humans need sleep, although some theories include energy conservation, restoration, and information processing. Sleep deprivation has many deleterious health effects. Residency programs have enacted strict work restrictions because of medically related errors due to sleep deprivation. Because obstetrics is an unpredictable specialty with long irregular hours, enacting a hospitalist program enhances patient safety, decreases malpractice risk, and improves the physician's quality of life by allowing obstetricians to get sufficient rest.

The concept of having an in-house obstetrician (serving as an obstetrics [OB] hospitalist) available 24 hours a day, 7 days a week provides a safety net for OB events that many need immediate intervention for a successful outcome. A key precept of risk management, that of loss prevention, fits perfectly with the addition of an OB hospitalist role in the perinatal department. Inherent in the role of OB hospitalists are the patient safety and risk management principles of improved communication, enhanced readiness, and immediate availability.

The thoughtful development and implementation of a comprehensive obstetric/gynecologic (OB/GYN) hospitalist program can result in a cost-effective practice model that provides increased value through a wide variety of services. The continuous on-site availability of an OB/GYN specialist affords many benefits to patients, hospitals, and practicing physicians. A well-implemented and effective OB/GYN hospitalist program will be associated with many different service line improvements for hospitals. Such programs increase patient safety, promote risk reduction, and improve clinical outcomes, while enriching the quality of life of obstetricians and gynecologists.

The growth of obstetric and gynecologic (OB/GYN) hospitalists throughout the United States has led to different organizational approaches, depending on the perception of what an OB/GYN hospitalist is. There are advantages of OB/GYN hospitalist practices; however, practitioners who do this as just 1 piece of their practice are not fulfilling the promise of what this new specialty can deliver. Because those with office practices have their own business models, this article is devoted to the organizational and business models of OB/GYN hospitalists for physicians whose practice is devoted to inpatient obstetrics with or without emergency room and/or inpatient gynecology coverage.

This article establishes the rationale and development of an obstetrics and gynecology (OB/GYN) hospitalist fellowship program. The pool of OB/GYN hospitalists needs to be drastically expanded to accommodate the country's needs. Fellowship programs should provide extra training and confidence for recent resident graduates who want to pursue a hospitalist career. Fellowships should train physicians in a way that aligns their interests with those of the hospital with respect to patient care, teaching, and research. Research in the core measures should be a necessary component of the fellowship so as to provide long-term benefits for all stakeholders, including hospitals and patients.

OBSTETRICS AND GYNECOLOGY CLINICS

THE CLINICS ARE AVAILABLE ONLINE!
Access your subscription at:
www.theclinics.com

Foreword

The Ob/Gyn Hospitalist: An Expanding Area of Practice Deserving Our Attention

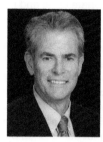

William F. Rayburn, MD, MBA
Consulting Editor

More than one year ago, I had the pleasure of listening to Dr Brigid McCue and Dr Jennifer Tessmer-Tuck lecture about an update about the Ob/Gyn Hospitalist—the present state and future. Their enthusiasm led me to approach them to guest edit an issue on this subject for the *Obstetrics and Gynecology Clinics of North America*. Their positive response was tempered by the need for assistance in preparing an issue to be best suited for the readership. Their effort in completing this task has led to a unique and valuable contribution to our very limited literature on the subject.

Hospital medicine is a medical specialty dedicated to the delivery of comprehensive care to hospitalized patients. Practitioners of hospital medicine include physicians (known as hospitalists) and nonphysician providers who engage in patient care, teaching, research, and leadership in the field of hospital medicine. In addition to their core expertise in managing the medical and surgical needs of acutely ill, hospitalized patients, hospitalists work to enhance the performance of hospitals and health care systems by prompting immediate attention to those patients when attention is sought, employing quality and process improvement techniques, collaborating with appropriate health workers, communicating and coordinating with all physicians and health care personnel, transitioning patient care safely within the hospital or to the community, and using resources responsibly.

The editors introduce the reader to what has transpired over the last two decades with care of hospitalized patients with the introduction of hospitalists, who consist of general internists, general pediatricians, and family physicians. Their challenges were and continue to be to improve population health, enhance the patient experience, and reduce per capita cost. What was learned from their experience and the impact to date on addressing these aims are addressed in this issue. Evolution of the Ob/Gyn

Obstet Gynecol Clin N Am 42 (2015) xiii–xiv
http://dx.doi.org/10.1016/j.ogc.2015.06.002
0889-8545/15/$ – see front matter © 2015 Published by Elsevier Inc.

hospitalist in the past decade has led to more refinements and opportunities to now measure the added benefits offered by their services to fellow Ob/Gyn practitioners and to hospitals.

This issue provides an excellent summary of activities relevant to practice settings in the labor and delivery suite, patient wards, operating room, emergency room, and inpatient clinics if available. The many authors represent experts in inpatient obstetrics, hospital medicine, quality improvement and patient safety, and business development. This issue permits the reader to have a much clearer understanding as to how the Ob/Gyn hospitalist practices to foster teamwork, coordinate care, and maximize efficiency. Their roles in assisting other Ob/Gyns with work-life balance is especially worthy of our attention.

The editors attempt at the issue's end to describe the future of Ob/Gyn hospital medicine. My suspicion is that the future will remain promising, since most Ob/Gyn practitioners work in urban locations in larger practices with the movement being toward more separate care at either outpatient or inpatient settings. Following residency training, Ob/Gyn graduates interested in additional learning opportunities will deal with the business of hospital medicine to acquire more expertise. Recognition of focused practice in Ob/Gyn hospital medicine will likely be aligned with that established by the American Board of Internal Medicine.

I appreciate the efforts by Dr McCue, Dr Tessmer-Tuck, and the many authors in shining light on this developing area of special clinical interest. The topics addressed in this issue incorporate priorities—quality and safe care, collaboration and communication, bridging between the hospital and community—that form essential components of contemporary women's health care.

William F. Rayburn, MD, MBA
Continuing Medical Education and Professional Development
Obstetrics and Gynecology
University of New Mexico School of Medicine
MSC 10 5580
1 University of New Mexico
Albuquerque, NM 87131-0001, USA

E-mail address:
wrayburn@salud.unm.edu

Preface

Obstetric and Gynecologic Hospitalists and Laborists

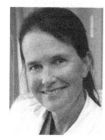 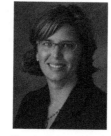

Brigid McCue, MD, PhD   Jennifer A. Tessmer-Tuck, MD
Editors

The Institute for Healthcare Improvement Triple Aim challenges us to improve the US health care system by addressing three objectives: improving population health, enhancing patient experience, and reducing per capita cost. Recently, some have called for the addition of "improving the work life health of health care providers," thereby making the Triple Aim a Quadruple Aim. Nowhere is the drive and ambition to achieve the Quadruple Aim more apparent than in the development and growth of OB/GYN Hospitalist medicine.

Over the last 20 years, care of hospitalized patients in the United States has been transformed by the introduction of hospitalists, physicians who dedicate their practice to caring for inpatients. These hospitalist physicians successfully partner with hospitals to meet the Triple Aim in notable areas, such as prevention of venous thromboembolic events and improvement of care coordination and care transitions. OB/GYN Hospitalist medicine initially evolved from similar needs to improve the quality and safety of care for hospitalized women. At the same time, however, OB/GYN hospitalist programs also recognized and addressed a critical need for the specialty of Obstetrics and Gynecology to evolve and change how care is provided in order to improve the work-life health of physicians in a specialty that, traditionally, has demanded long work hours and time away from home and family.

This issue of *Obstetrics and Gynecology Clinics of North America* provides a summary of topics relevant to OB/GYN Hospitalist medicine. Multiple experts in the fields of inpatient obstetrics, hospital medicine, patient safety and quality improvement, and business development have contributed to the issue. What can we learn from the history of traditional internal medicine hospitalists and the impact they have had to date on addressing the Triple Aim? Like traditional hospitalists, evolving data suggest that OB/GYN Hospitalists can improve quality of care by reducing cesarean section rates and improving rates of vaginal birth after cesarean section. Are there other quality improvement opportunities? For example, can OB/GYN Hospitalists play a role in

Obstet Gynecol Clin N Am 42 (2015) xv–xvi
http://dx.doi.org/10.1016/j.ogc.2015.06.001
0889-8545/15/$ – see front matter © 2015 Published by Elsevier Inc.

helping to curb the rise in maternal morbidity and mortality in the United States and improve the overall safety of obstetrical care? How can you design your OB/GYN Hospitalist practice to maximize efficiency, teamwork, and coordination of care while simultaneously balancing these quality and safety improvements against provider work-life health? Ultimately, what is the future of OB/GYN Hospitalist medicine and will (should) it become its own boarded subspecialty with recognized fellowships?

Though 12 years have passed since Louis Weinstein first coined the term "Laborist," there is no doubt that OB/GYN Hospitalist medicine is in its infancy. It is our sincerest hope that, in years to come, the next OB/GYN Hospitalist issue of *Obstetrics and Gynecology Clinics of North America* is full of published evidence supporting OB/GYN Hospitalists and successfully achieving the Quadruple Aim to improve population health, enhance patient experience, and reduce per capita cost while improving the work-life health of all OB/GYN providers.

Brigid McCue, MD, PhD
Beth Israel Deaconess Hospital-Plymouth
275 Sandwich Street
Plymouth, MA 02360, USA

Jennifer A. Tessmer-Tuck, MD
North Memorial Medical Center
3300 Oakdale Avenue North
Robbinsdale, MN 55422, USA

E-mail addresses:
bmccue@bidplymouth.org (B. McCue)
Jennifer.tessmertuck@gmail.com (J.A. Tessmer-Tuck)

Laborist to Obstetrician/ Gynecologist–Hospitalist
An Evolution or a Revolution?

Louis Weinstein, MD

KEYWORDS

- Laborist • Hospitalist • Obstetrics • Gynecology

KEY POINTS

- A major advantage of a laborist/hospitalist program is the standardization of clinical care of the patient by developing evidence based protocols.
- The critical issue in any laborist/hospitalist program is the limitation of work hours for the physician, which has the potential to eliminate the problem of fatigue and decrease burnout.
- Having a laborist/hospitalist program allows the institution to always have a rapid response team for any emergent clinical condition.
- The laborist/hospitalist mode of practice is very conducive to the needs of the Generation X and Y physicians.

The first decade of the 21st century has resulted in many changes to the profession of obstetrics & gynecology. The explosion of knowledge, the introduction of new technology, and the ever-present, escalating professional liability insurance costs all impact the practicing obstetrician/gynecologist. Other changes include the plethora of subspecialists negatively impacting resident experience, the continuing decrease in the number of hours worked by residents, the marked increase in the use of minimally invasive surgical techniques including the introduction of robotic surgery, and most noticeably the marked gender shift in the field (the most rapid in the history of medicine), resulting in the overwhelming number of practitioners and trainees being female.[1] The most noticeable change in the profession has been the introduction of the importance of work–life balance by generation Y physicians (millennials). This is not gender driven, but rather generational, and is similar for both genders. This change will have the most profound long lasting impact on the profession because of the desire of the generation Y physicians to work fewer hours and to leave the practice of obstetrics at a much younger age, resulting in a continuing increase in the shortage of working obstetricians.

PO Box 21829, Charleston, SC 29413, USA
E-mail address: Louis.weinstein@jefferson.edu

Obstet Gynecol Clin N Am 42 (2015) 415–417
http://dx.doi.org/10.1016/j.ogc.2015.05.001
0889-8545/15/$ – see front matter © 2015 Elsevier Inc. All rights reserved.

obgyn.theclinics.com

It became obvious in the mid 1980s that many aspects related to the practice of obstetrics were not safe for either the patient or the physician.[2] There were too many errors occurring on the labor unit that were impacting both the mother and her unborn child. Physicians were working an excessive number of hours secondary to call requirements and often functioning at a level similar to that of an inebriated individual.[3] These issues suggested that a better system of practice for obstetrics needed to be developed. This resulted in my publication in 2003 that introduced the concept of the laborist as a new method of practice that had the potential to improve both patient safety and physician well-being.[4] The concept of the laborist was based on the model developed in 1996 by Wachter and Goldman of the hospitalist, a model that has become extremely prevalent and quite successful in the current practice of internal medicine.[5] After the first publication introducing the laborist as a practice model, there was little movement regarding its introduction into clinical practice.[4] As physician dissatisfaction and burnout in obstetrics and gynecology approached epidemic levels, however, laborists seemed to be a possible solution and programs began developing across the nation.[6,7]

The role of the laborist as initially envisioned was to care only for patients on the labor unit and to manage obstetric emergencies. The laborist was to function as a rapid response team and only manage the patient if the private practitioner chose to relinquish care. Also, the laborist was available to offer backup to the nurse midwife or the family practitioner practicing obstetrics. The advantages of the laborist are numerous. She or he is immediately available to the nurses to evaluate fetal monitoring, address dysfunctional labor, adjust oxytocin dosage, and for the unexpected obstetric emergency that requires an immediate decision regarding an intervention. The laborist is free of the stresses of a private practice, works a constant and controllable schedule, can have work shift limitations, thereby eliminating the issue of fatigue and impairment, and improve patient safety while decreasing the potential for adverse outcomes that may result in a liability action.

The establishment of a laborist program also allows an institution to develop evidence-based protocols for patient management, eliminating the common problem in obstetric practice of having practitioners using their autonomy in patient care that is often not evidenced based. The standardization of labor management, fetal monitor interpretation, and oxytocin administration will have a huge impact on the improvement of patient safety.

There are many advantages of the laborist to the private practitioner. The presence of the laborist allows the practitioner to continue to offer antepartum care while being relieved of the excessive time commitment of dealing with the laboring patient. Daily activities will be less stressful because the physician will not have to balance office hours or operating time with constant disruptions from labor and delivery. The obvious decrease in on-call time requirements will have the potential to improve work–lifestyle balance, dissatisfaction, and burnout. Medical legal risk will be decreased—the labor unit is the major source for adverse outcomes leading to an obstetric legal action.

There is potential for concern about patient dissatisfaction with having a laborist, who the patient may never have met, manage the labor process. When the role of the laborist is explained to the patient along with the fact that the physician is not fatigued and is only there to assist when needed, the acceptance of patients is extremely high. One report of 3 years of a laborist program revealed no patients complaints regarding the role of the laborist; another had 1 complaint among approximately 2400 obstetric patients.[8]

There are numerous models for laborist programs and each institution has the ability to establish a program that is best suited to their individual needs. A survey of obstetric/gynecologic hospitalists and laborists revealed the biggest variation difference occurred in the number of hours worked per shift.[9] As I originally proposed, a laborist would not work more than a 14-hour shift, because fatigue and impairment markedly increase when the shift exceeds 16 consecutive hours.[4] If the 2 major goals of a laborist program are to improve patient safety and physician well-being, then the number of hours worked must be controlled. The same survey revealed that the median number of actual hours worked per shift was 16, with a 24-hour shift length being the one most commonly reported.[9] The report demonstrated that the majority of hospitals also allowed the laborist to work outside their main site (moonlight). If the goals of this practice model are to improve patient safety and physician well-being, these issues need to be addressed and controlled. One could argue that the maximum length of a laborist shift should be 16 hours, with the ideal for each day having 2 laborists with one working 10 hours and the other 14 hours. The contract between the institution and the laborist should not allow additional outside work (moonlighting), because this allows the individual to work excessive number of hours, defeating one of the major reasons to establish a laborist program. This type of control works best when the laborist is employed by the institution and has a signed contract delineating all the specifics of employment. As related to career satisfaction, the same study revealed a high career satisfaction rate among the laborist and obstetric/gynecologic hospitalists.[9] The major reason cited for the high level of satisfaction was the ability to control the schedule along with its constancy.

The laborist model offers the best approach to standardize care and improve patient safety on the labor unit, improve physician well-being, and decrease physician dissatisfaction/burnout. This is what is being demanded both by patients and generation Y physicians. It is time to recognize the importance of the laborist to our profession because she or he can be "just what the Doctor has ordered."

REFERENCES

1. Weinstein L. Where have all the young men gone. Ob Gyn Management 2011;23: 10–2.
2. Weinstein L. Malpractice - the syndrome of the 80's. Obstet Gynecol 1988;72: 130–5.
3. Weinstein L, Garite T. On call for obstetrics – time for a change. Am J Obstet Gynecol 2007;196:3.
4. Weinstein L. The Laborist - a new focus of practice for the obstetrician. Am J Obstet Gynecol 2003;188:310–2.
5. Wachter RM, Goldman L. The emerging role of "hospitalists" in the American health care system. N Engl J Med 1996;335:514–7.
6. Weinstein L, Wolfe HM. The downward spiral of physician satisfaction – an attempt to avert a crisis within the medical profession. Obstet Gynecol 2007;109:1181–3.
7. Weinstein L. The unbearable unhappiness of the ObGyn: a crisis looms. Ob Gyn Management 2008;20:34–42.
8. Gussman D, Mann W. The laborists: a flexible concept. Washington, DC: American College of Obstetricians and Gynecologists; 2007.
9. Funk C, Anderson BL, Schulkin J, et al. Survey of obstetric and gynecologic hospitalists and laborists. Am J Obstet Gynecol 2010;203:177.e1–4.

A History of the Hospitalist Movement

Jordan Messler, MD, SFHM[a],*, Winthrop F. Whitcomb, MD, MHM[b]

KEYWORDS

- Hospitalists • Hospital medicine • Laborists • Hospital-focused specialties
- History of hospitalists • Patient safety

KEY POINTS

- Hospitalists emerged as a new practice pattern in the 1990s in the face of a changing health care financial landscape, primary care physicians (PCPs) leaving the hospital, and a push to improve the efficiency and effectiveness of hospital care.
- One of the early successes for hospital medicine was centering its mission on a quality and patient safety agenda.
- Hospital-focused specialties, such as obstetrics and gynecology (OBGYN) hospitalists, are emerging rapidly. The success of these specialists depends on various strategies, including aligning with hospital goals, creating a clear research agenda, adapting to the changing health care financial landscape, and pursuing a mission to improve patient safety and the quality of care in the hospital.

INTRODUCTION

Hospital medicine has grown from a physician specialty that did not exist in name 20 years ago to a burgeoning field of over 48,000 hospitalists[1] practicing in almost 80% of US hospitals[1] with one-third of Medicare admissions being under a hospitalist's care.[2] One of the latest and fastest growing fields in medicine emerged in an environment of changing health care finances, increased flight of PCPs from the hospital, and a growing patient safety need for 24/7 physician coverage in the hospital. Further growth was fueled by the need for better physician alignment with the hospital, resident work hour restrictions, the regulatory focus on quality and patient safety, and the increasing complexity of care for the hospitalized patient. The value of this growth has been borne out in improved quality metrics, efficiency, and cost savings. The history of the hospitalist movement has been well covered by Wachter[3,4] along

Disclosures: The authors have nothing to disclose.
[a] Incompass Health, Morton Plant Hospital, 300 Pinellas Street, #47, Clearwater, FL 33756, USA;
[b] Remedy Partners, 1120 Post Road, Darien, CT 06820, USA
* Corresponding author.
E-mail address: Jordan.messler@baycare.org

Obstet Gynecol Clin N Am 42 (2015) 419–432
http://dx.doi.org/10.1016/j.ogc.2015.05.002
0889-8545/15/$ – see front matter © 2015 Elsevier Inc. All rights reserved.

obgyn.theclinics.com

with Goldman[5] in a series of articles over the years. This article reexamines this history and attempts to align with the growth of OBGYN hospitalists.

OBGYN hospitalists are at a similar point today at which hospital medicine was in the late 1990s. The OBGYN hospitalist model was first proposed in 2003, and by 2010, it was estimated that 40% of US hospitals were using OBGYN hospitalists.[6] Peeling back the drivers, challenges, and successes of hospital medicine may help OBGYN hospitalists and other hospital-focused specialists prepare for their growth.

EARLY HISTORY OF HOSPITALISTS

Variations of physicians in the hospital setting existed for centuries. On Tiber Island, in Rome, is one of the oldest sites of medical care, with the establishment of an Aesculapian temple in 293 BC. Aesculapian temples are some of the earliest representations of hospitals, and the Aesculapian priests who worked there were theoretically the first hospitalists. Practitioners of medicine had minimal diagnostic or therapeutics until the nineteenth century. The modern physician evolved once a more careful physical examination was possible, as one of many key steps was Laennec's discovery of the stethoscope in 1815. By the end of the nineteenth century, the hospital as we know it today began to emerge, and particularly emblematic was the opening of The Johns Hopkins Hospital in 1889. The combination of clinical faculty, research, and education modernized medical care. Teaching and clinical medicine were born, and the hospitalist model had its modern icon in Osler. Soon after, Ernest Codman in Boston pioneered ideas about hospital standards and incorporated scientific management ideas into hospital quality and safety efforts. By the end of the twentieth century, all these elements would coalesce into the modern hospitalist movement.

MODERN HISTORY OF HOSPITALISTS

Before the era of hospitalists, traditional physicians (whether an internist, obstetrician, or other specialist) often visited the hospital in the morning, saw their office patients, and ended their day with a return to the hospital to see patients (**Box 1**). Weekends were spent covering more than 1 hospital, and the schedule consisted of frequent night calls. In the 1970s, PCPs spent almost half of their clinical time in the hospital, with about 10 patients to see daily during rounds. Internists' inpatient load steadily reduced. By the early 1990s, internists saw about 2 patients per day in the hospital and spent less than 10% of their time on hospital care.[7] The lengthy days, the lack of availability for hospital emergencies, the numerous office interruptions, and the impact on revenue convinced many internists to focus on the office.

Although many physicians left the hospital, a small cadre focused their care in the hospital. By 1994, 10% of internists and 4% of family practitioners dedicated more than 50% of their time to the hospital setting.[8] During this time, several models of hospital medicine in the United States emerged. These models have been discussed in detail elsewhere.[9,10] In California, in 1994, inpatient managers were created to help improve inpatient care. This Kaiser Permanente model emerged out of the managed care environment. Park Nicollet in Minnesota established similar models.[11] The goals of these models were to improve quality, focus on patient-centered care, and improve patient satisfaction.[12] These models sought the same changes that hospital medicine groups seek today: to minimize unnecessary admissions and disruptions in the outpatient clinic from hospital calls, to effect a timely hospital discharge, to avoid unnecessary consults, and to reduce physician burnout. The outpatient physicians as per this model were seeing on an average 1 inpatient a day, contributing to inefficient care.[12]

Box 1
Important dates in the history of hospital medicine

History of recent hospital medicine

- 1980s and early 1990s: Protohospitalist models reported in various locales around the United States
- 1994: Inpatient managers in California, Minneapolis, and elsewhere, cover PCP patients in the hospital
- August 1996: Wachter and Goldman name hospitalists
- October 1996: Nelson and Whitcomb begin developing NAIP
- March 1997: *The Hospitalist*—the first publication devoted to hospital medicine—is published
- April 1997: The first hospital medicine conference takes place in San Francisco
- July 1997: NAIP incorporated
- April 1998: NAIP opens membership and holds first annual meeting
- 2003: NAIP changes names to SHM
- 2004: 10,000 hospitalists nationally
- 2006: *Journal of Hospital Medicine* first published
- 2006: Hospital medicine core competencies published
- 2008: Project BOOST, SHM-mentored implementation program
- 2010: ABIM creates Recognition of Focused Practice in Hospital Medicine
- 2011: Eisenberg Award for SHM: mentored implementation award
- 2014: 48,000 hospitalists nationally

Abbreviations: ABIM, American Board of Internal Medicine; NAIP, National Association of Inpatient Physicians; SHM, Society of Hospital Medicine.

In 1996, Wachter and Goldman published a piece in the *New England Journal of Medicine* naming physicians dedicated to inpatient care as hospitalists.[12] Hospitalists were initially defined people who spend more than 25% of their clinical time in the hospital. At present, the Society of Hospital Medicine (SHM) definition broadly states that a hospitalist is a "physician who specializes in the practice of hospital medicine."[13] The generally accepted definition is a physician with a primary focus in caring for the hospitalized patient. SHM defines hospital medicine as "a medical specialty dedicated to the delivery of comprehensive medical care to hospitalized patients."[13] The Society of OBGYN Hospitalists (SOGH) defines an OBGYN hospitalist as "An Obstetrician/Gynecologist who has focused their professional practice on care of the hospitalized woman." The term *laborist* is frequently used in reference to OBGYN hospitalists, and SOGH defines this practitioner as "An Obstetrician/Gynecologist who has focused their professional practice on the care of women in Labor and Delivery."[14]

The naming started a movement, with the elements of a society and a specialty emerging from hospital medicine's first leaders: Wachter, John Nelson, and Win Whitcomb. After seeing the 1996 article, Nelson and Whitcomb reached out to Wachter to build a home for hospital medicine; they discussed a gathering of self-identified hospitalists, and the first official hospital medicine meeting took place in San Francisco in April 1997. Nelson and Whitcomb assembled a board of directors and sought the creation of a new society for hospitalists. The first version of the society was the National

Association of Inpatient Physicians (NAIP). Nelson and Whitcomb were the founders and first copresidents; they added members formally on April 1, 1998, the same date as the first annual meeting of NAIP. By 2002, NAIP had 1800 members and there were 4500 hospitalists nationally. NAIP started in affiliation with the American College of Physicians (ACP), which meant that NAIP would use selected ACP resources but would remain an independent society. In 2003, NAIP changed names to the SHM. SHM understands the importance of helping young societies grow and today helps provide basic infrastructure support for the SOGH.

After NAIP was incorporated in July 1997, one of the first committees specified on the organizational chart was the ethics committee. This committee saw the importance[15] of creating a framework that helped define a new field in medicine that kept the interests of the patient front and center. This ethical framework was tested early on, as several managed care companies were looking to mandate referral to hospitalists by PCPs, presumably because hospitalists were thought to provide less-costly hospital care. NAIP's first formal position was to state that these referrals be voluntary, left to the discretion of the physicians and their patients. Within a short time, 2 dozen other medical societies adopted similar positions. This adoption led most managed care companies to abandon the compulsory referral to hospitalists for inpatient care.[16]

A crucial decision from the society's inception was to welcome the involvement of all members of the hospital team in advancing the specialty. Hospital medicine became an inclusionary group, not separating academic or community spheres, adding pediatricians, and being sure to include family practitioners and advanced practice providers (APPs). NAIP espoused a big tent philosophy for those dedicated to improving the care of patients in the hospital and built an array of committees, educational offerings, workgroups, and other resources to support interdisciplinary, team-based care.

Early steps by academic leaders set to codify the knowledge of hospital medicine, with textbooks soon published.[17–20] *The Hospitalist* was the first publication devoted entirely to hospital medicine, leading the way for the *Journal of Hospital Medicine* (JHM). The JHM is a peer-reviewed journal geared for hospitalists and supported hospital medicine research publication, a critical element in building a specialty. In 2006, the core competencies were published to help define the skill set and associated educational and teaching aspects of hospital medicine.[21]

As hospital medicine grew, a certification that recognized unique expertise in hospital medicine was established. In 2010, the American Board of Internal Medicine rolled out Recognition of Focused Practice in Hospital Medicine[22]; this consists of a secure examination and a series of practice improvement modules aimed at recognizing quality improvement initiatives and was launched as a pathway for general internists to earn Maintenance of Certification in Internal Medicine. This pathway was also made available to family physicians.

EARLY CHALLENGES AND SOLUTIONS

The steady growth was not without challenges. Hospitalists faced backlash from hospitals and PCPs who were not sure of these new physicians invading their turf. Editorials bemoaned the death knell of quality care for patients in the hospital and loss of continuity of care as patients transitioned into or out of the hospital.[23,24] Other concerns, such as the fear that hospitalists would steal patients from PCPs, proved to be groundless.

What overcame many of these challenges, and perhaps a central element of hospital medicine's growth, was its call to quality and patient safety. Hospital medicine's leadership seized on the message of the first Institute Of Medicine Report, "To Err is Human: Building a Safer Health System"[25] in 1999, and the estimated 44,000 to 98,000 annual avoidable deaths in American hospitals.[26] Soon after, quality and patient safety were discussed as a critical focus for the field by several of its leaders.[27,28] Quality became the central vision for SHM and hospitalists. By 2010, SHM created a Center for Hospital Innovation and Improvement to further hospitalists' mission for quality. The SHM sought to develop future leaders through its Leadership Academy and Mentor University. For its mentoring work in quality improvement projects, SHM won the Eisenberg Award, recognizing outstanding contribution to quality of patient care, the first medical society to win this award.[29]

Growth of Hospital Medicine/Drivers of Hospital Medicine

Hospital medicine grew rapidly. From 1995 to 2006, the number of internal medicine physicians who identified themselves as hospitalists increased 4-fold (from 5% to 19%).[30] By 2007, there were 20,000 hospitalists in the United States, and today, there are over 40,000. In 2007, 29% of all US hospitals, and 55% hospitals with more than 500 beds, had hospitalists.[1,31]

Why did hospital medicine grow so quickly? The field originated largely because of practice patterns, the desire for primary physicians to focus on the clinic, and the imperative to develop a system for the focused care of inpatients. In addition, care became more fragmented in the hospital, with specialists driving the care and lack of a clear captain of the ship. Health care financial drivers also helped accelerate the growth. As Medicare shifted to diagnosis-related groups (DRG) payments in the 1980s, incentives existed for hospitals to lower length of stay, which created pressure for physicians to provide efficient hospital care. In addition, many PCPs were happy to leave the hospital, to both avoid the discontinuity in their day by coming to the hospital before and after clinic and the barrage of hospital nursing calls during clinic hours. Hospitals looked to hospitalists for solutions to these ubiquitous challenges.

More recent drivers include residency work hour changes, increased acuity of inpatients, and further demands on PCPs. ACGME (Accreditation Council for Graduate Medical Education) work hours began capping residents at 80 hours in 2003[32]; this led many academic hospitalist groups to add nonteaching services to offload residents and teaching teams. In addition, hospitalists were available to provide 24/7 in-hospital coverage and improve day-to-day teaching and training.[33]

The increased comorbidities of inpatients demanded physicians who were dedicated to inpatient care.[34] PCPs continued to face time constraints, needing to see more patients in a shorter time frame. PCPs also received reduced reimbursements, so that eliminating hospital duties was a way to save time and increase revenue in the office.[35] Other specialists became more inclined to have the ever-available hospitalist admit their patients; hospitalists began admitting many primary surgical admissions.[36] Overall, these drivers created a continued need for an inpatient manager of care: the hospitalist.

CURRENT STATE OF HOSPITAL MEDICINE

Hospitalists are present in over 90% of hospitals with 200 or more beds.[1] Hospitalists have grown 10-fold from 2000 to today; they are ubiquitous in major hospitals and in almost all teaching hospitals. As of 2014, there are 48,000 hospitalists[1] and 12,000 members in SHM (**Fig. 1**).

Individual hospitalist groups vary; a common refrain being, "if you've seen one hospitalist group, you've seen one hospitalist group." The 2014 State of Hospital Medicine report, consisting of 2013 survey data from SHM and medical group management association (MGMA), provides a snapshot of hospital medicine today.[37] Almost

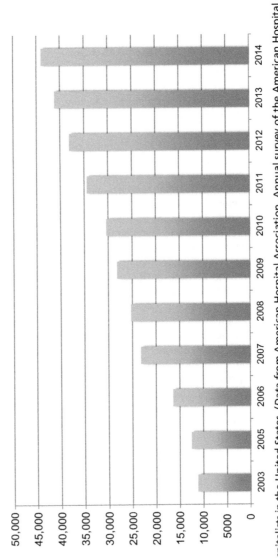

Fig. 1. Growth of hospitalists in the United States. (*Data from* American Hospital Association. Annual survey of the American Hospital Association. Chicago: American Hospital Association; 2013.)

half of the hospitalist groups surveyed were used by a hospital or health care delivery system. One-third of the hospitalist groups existed for less than 5 years, and 10% existed for more than 15 years. Arrangements with hospitalists are variable. About 50% of hospitals or health care systems use their hospitalists. Other arrangements may include management companies used by hospitals to maintain the group, private multispecialty or primary care groups, or private-hospitalist-only medical groups.

There are many ways to create the hospitalist schedule. Most groups (54%) use 7-on-7-off scheduling blocks, and 10.4% use another type of rotating block. Few groups use a Monday through Friday schedule. As one of the main benefits of hospitalists is a 24/7 presence, it is consistent that over 80% of groups have a hospitalist available in-house overnight. Changes are made because of local culture, volumes, and physician preference (**Table 1**).

What Do Hospitalists Do Today?

The vast majority of hospitalist work remains clinical patient duties, yet many other opportunities exist in the hospital (**Table 2**).[38] Hospitalists are actively involved in comanagement with surgical services, particularly orthopedics.[39] Some hospitalist groups divide up services among nocturnists (those working exclusively at night, with either more pay or less shifts to compensate for the more arduous shifts). Other hospitalists serve as the intensivists for a hospital. Hospitalists run observation units and short-stay units, oversee code teams, or help coordinate rapid response teams. About 15% of hospitalist groups do palliative care work[40] (see **Table 2** to outline other areas that hospitalists find ways to engage in the hospital outside of clinical work).

As their presence in the hospital grows, OBGYN hospitalists will also find new opportunities to improve quality, lead, and engage in the hospital.

OUTCOMES
Research Providing Evidence of Hospital Medicine Effectiveness

One of the earliest challenges for hospitalists was demonstrating their value, proving that implementing a 24/7 hospitalist model would translate into real value for the

Table 1 Various types of hospitalist scheduling models	
Hospitalist Scheduling Models	**%**
Shift work	85
Variable	12
Call	2
Other	1
Nocturnists	58
Backup call	58
7-on-7-off	54
Other block shifts	10
Monday-Friday	4
Variable	29
Other	3

Data from Society of Hospital Medicine. 2014 State of Hospital medicine report. Available at: www.hospitalmedicine.org/survey2014. Accessed February 9, 2015.

Table 2 Roles for hospitalists	
Clinical	Comanagement
	Consultative
	Preoperative care
	Postdischarge clinic
	Skilled nursing facilities
	Critical care areas
	Inpatient wards
	Palliative care
Educational	Academic teaching service
	Clerkship director
	Curriculum development
	Residency program director
Quality	Quality officer
	Patient safety officer
	Quality educator
Operational	Bed flow coordination
	Utilization management
Information technology	EMR implementation
Research	Clinical research, QI research
Administrative	Quality officers
	Chief medical officers
	Other leadership positions

Abbreviations: EMR, electronic medical record; QI, quality improvement.
Adapted from Sehgal NL. The expanding role of hospitalists in the United States. Swiss Med Wkly 2006;136:591.

investment in people and resources. Early data supported length of stay reduction in an academic hospitalist group.[41] Others also reported lower lengths of stay in other settings, translating into clear cost savings.[39,42–44]

Readmissions have been shown to stay the same or decrease with hospitalist care.[45] Hospitalists adhere to guidelines,[46–48] improve quality of care,[44] and increase patient satisfaction.[49]

Most data supporting hospitalists are positive, but other studies raise important questions. For instance, many studies are single-site studies and perhaps not generalizable.[42] Some of the reported improved outcomes associated with hospitalists are afflicted with poor methodology.[50] Also, hospitalists may decrease hospital stay costs, but possibly at the expense of increased postacute care costs.[51,52] In addition, hospitalists are not necessarily independent factors in improving patient quality[53]; this is consistent with the notion that hospitals are complex, and although the use of hospitalists is a structure of care change, improvements in quality are caused by the interplay of a myriad of factors.[25]

The quality and patient safety initiatives that hospitalists work on remain their calling card. SHM has prepared many models of improvement, with resource rooms, improvement plans, and mentorship for such areas as transitions of care (Project BOOST [Better Outcomes by Optimizing Safe Transitions]), thromboembolism prevention, and diabetes care.[54] Hospitalists also understood early on that they were the source of the "voltage drop" of information from hospital discharge to PCP follow-up. One of the earliest systematic quality improvement projects that SHM created to mentor other hospitals on care improvement was around care transitions. Project BOOST, created in

2008, is a multidisciplinary approach to offer solutions in reducing the transitional care gap.[55] (see article by Howell elsewhere in this issue to further understand how hospitalists have been working to improve quality and patient safety in the hospital setting).

COMMON ISSUES FACING HOSPITAL MEDICINE TODAY AND POTENTIAL SOLUTIONS

Hospitalists currently find themselves in a coveted position: a rapidly growing field, with many opportunities for growth in both care delivery and leadership roles and testing frequent care innovations. However, many challenges face hospitalists today that may face OBGYN hospitalists as their field grows,[56] including physician burnout, financial stability, and workforce shortages.

Hospitalists are concerned about burnout in their field, working in a highly stressful 7-day, shift-based schedule, with frequent night rotations and increasing censuses. Burnout can lead to unprofessional behavior, loss of effectiveness, and a cynical outlook on medicine. Hospitalists do not seem to experience more burnout than outpatient physicians,[57] but burnout and work-life balance are important aspects of hospitalists' work.[58] Part of this burnout may be remedied by making adjustments in scheduling. Finding the right schedule model and the sweet spot for daily census volume bedevils every hospitalist medical director; it is individualized to a group and depends on a variety of local patterns. For instance, questions such as are hospitalists also functioning as the intensivists, what is the unassigned patient percentage, and how much support is there from APPs and other professionals and many other questions should play a role in determining ideal volumes and patient load. In addition, groups often decide whether they should have surge protection for unexpected volume shifts. Hospitalist leaders take all this into account, knowing that an increasing workload may increase length of stay (in addition to burnout).[59] OBGYN hospitalists decide which variables to take into account to determine the right scheduling model and census load.

Most hospital medicine groups require subsidies from hospitals to meet practice expenses, most of which is salary and benefits. These subsidies have been steadily increasing and are an important part of the stability for hospital medicine groups. Hospitalist groups continually have to justify this support, either through quality work or through financial measures or other supporting roles. OBGYN hospitalists, to provide 24/7 care, may also require subsidies, depending on their care model.[60]

In a rapidly growing specialty such as hospital medicine, it is a real concern that demand will outpace the supply of qualified practitioners. A solution for workload management is the use of APPs. The number of APPs in hospital medicine continues to grow,[37] because they can be effective and efficient additions to hospitals medicine groups.[33,61]

In 2005, turnover was about 13% per year, while the latest survey data put that number about the same, at 14%.[60]

OBGYN hospitalists will likely face some of these same challenges. In addition, they will face some of the other early challenges hospitalists have faced, such as maintaining good relationships and communication with their outpatient colleagues. Patients will question why they are not seeing their own obstetrician in the hospital. Continuous presence in the hospital and a focus on the hospitalized patient without a competing clinic are likely what help keep hospitalist patient satisfaction scores better or comparable to PCPs and will probably do the same for OBGYN hospitalists.

FUTURE OF HOSPITAL MEDICINE

The future of hospital medicine will depend on how hospitalists respond to issues such as the rapid growth of the specialty, changes in health payment reform, and new modes of health care delivery such as accountable care organizations (ACOs) and bundled payments.

Value-based purchasing may fundamentally alter the health care landscape. As payments grow to cover extended periods, such as 30- or 90-day episodes, and not just the hospital stay, care management will change. Hospitalists will be working more closely with PCPs, home care providers, and postdischarge facilities caring for their hospitalized patients. The need to more rigorously select the appropriate, value-based site of care after hospital discharge will grow in successful bundled payment programs and ACOs. More models may emerge, such as the back to basics model of Meltzer. His Comprehensive Care Physician model studies hospitalists caring for some of their more complex patients longitudinally like a traditional internist.[62] Other solutions include postdischarge clinics.[63,64]

ACOs may also change how care is managed and how hospitalists practice. In the 2014 State of Hospital Medicine survey, 35.8% of hospitalist groups were "involved or considering involvement with ACOs."[60] In moving toward better population health management, PCPs, hospitalists, and other postacute care providers and facilities will need to improve care coordination. Better transfer of information and safer management of patients between health care settings will necessarily emerge.

In addition, hospitalists are continuing to innovate and build upon care models. For instance, efforts by hospitalists have resulted in improved teamwork in the hospital, by localizing physicians to units,[65] creating clear roles and goals for teams in patient-centered care,[66,67] and partnering with nursing/nurse directors on units.[68]

HOSPITAL-FOCUSED SPECIALTIES

As hospitalists grow, so do new fields in hospital medicine. Hospital-focused specialties have existed before hospitalists, with critical-care-based pulmonologists and many other specialties doing most of their work in the hospital; this is becoming more codified and resembles the early days of hospital medicine. Emerging fields in this area include neurohospitalists, surgicalists, and OBGYN hospitalists. In the 2014 SHM survey, the following patterns were seen in hospitals with hospital-focused practices: 35% of hospitals had hospital-based intensivists; 16.6% in general surgery, 9.6% with OB/GYN, 15.7% with neurology, 7.2% with gastrointestinal tract/liver, 8.2% with cardiology, 5.6% with orthopedics, and 10.1% with hospital-based psychiatrists.[60] These hospital-focused specialties may continue to grow as hospitals use more physicians and require a dedicated group of practitioners of care to effect change. In addition, the growth will be driven by efforts to improve practice patterns for physicians.

OBSTETRICS AND GYNECOLOGY HOSPITALIST MODEL

The OBGYN hospitalist model will see many of the same drivers, challenges, and models that emerged in hospital medicine. OBGYN hospitalists are a rapidly emerging field, currently instituting a new infrastructure, with competencies, scheduling, related outcomes, and a clear research agenda. The growth and challenges of hospital medicine can provide lessons to help OBGYN hospitalists develop into a bona fide specialty.[69]

OBGYN hospitalists will face challenges from patients who want to see their own obstetrician in-hospital. Offering the advantages of 24/7, on-site presence will mitigate these challenges. OBGYN hospitalists will also work alongside physicians who do not want to give up inpatient care for the foreseeable future. Various models of care will emerge, driven by local needs and cultural factors. Hospitals will be committed to the success of the OBGYN hospitalists model if both the quality and financial metrics favor it.

The growth of the OBGYN hospitalist model needs to parallel a commitment to quality, patient safety, education, and outcomes research. The field will succeed if it focuses on creating better systems of care. The science of quality improvement and patient safety creates enormous potential for OBGYN hospitalists in both academic and community hospital settings.

SUMMARY

About 10 years of OBGYN hospitalists, 20 years of hospitalists, almost 200 years of the modern hospital, and over 2000 thousand years of practitioners in hospital-like entities have been witnessed. The care for the patient is the constant throughout time. As the acuity of hospitalized patients has increased over time, the need for specialization in hospital care has grown, with a corresponding rise in the number and variety of physicians practicing solely in the hospital. The dramatic growth in the number of hospitalists over the past 20 years has been driven by many factors, such as physician practice patterns, financial drivers, and hospital quality improvement needs. The early establishment of key elements of a specialty, such as a professional society, and the emerging patient safety movement, helped define hospitalists and drive their mission. OBGYN hospitalists are in a similar position to effect change in the hospital, driving better processes and clinical outcomes, within the right structural model.

Much of the promise of the emerging hospital-focused specialties lies in their natural focus on systems of care, with a great potential to improve quality and efficiency. As more colleagues are dedicated to hospital care, there will be a need for better collaboration within the hospital and between hospital and clinic. As such collaborative care grows, this will likely translate into a safer health care system, with better outcomes for all patients.

REFERENCES

1. American Hospital Association. Annual survey of the American Hospital Association. Chicago: American Hospital Association; 2013.
2. Pete Welch W, Stearns SC, Cuellar AE, et al. Use of hospitalists by Medicare beneficiaries: a national picture. Medicare Medicaid Res Rev 2014;4(2). http://dx.doi.org/10.5600/mmrr2014-004-02-b01.
3. Wachter RM. The evolution of the hospitalist model in the United States. Med Clin North Am 2002;86(4):687–706.
4. Wachter RM. The state of hospital medicine in 2008. Med Clinic North Am 2008;92(2):265–73.
5. Wachter RM, Goldman L. The hospitalist movement 5 years later. JAMA 2002;287(4):487–94.
6. Srinivas SK, Shocksnider J, Caldwell D, et al. Laborist model of care: who is using it? J Matern Fetal Neonatal Med 2012;25(3):257–60.
7. Wachter RM. Response to David Meltzer's paper, "Hospitalists and the doctor-patient relationship". J Legal Stud 2001;30(2):615–23.
8. Saint S, Christakis DA, Baldwin LM, et al. Is hospitalism new? An analysis of medicare data from Washington State in 1994. Eff Clin Pract 2000;3(1):35–9.
9. Wachter RM. Reflections: the hospitalist movement a decade later. J Hosp Med 2006;1(4):248–52.
10. Craig DE, Hartka L, Likosky WH, et al. Implementation of a hospitalist system in a large health maintenance organization: the Kaiser Permanente experience. Ann Intern Med 1999;130(4 Pt 2):355–9.

11. Freese RB. The Park Nicollet experience in establishing a hospitalist system. Ann Intern Med 1999;130(4 Pt 2):350–4.

12. Wachter RM, Goldman L. The emerging role of "hospitalists" in the American health care system. N Engl J Med 1996;335(7):514–7.

13. Society of Hospital Medicine. About SHM. Available at: www.hospitalmedicine.org/Web/About_SHM/Industry/Hospital_Medicine_Hospital_Definition.aspx. Accessed February 1, 2015.

14. Available at: http://www.societyofobgynhospitalists.com/scriptcontent/index.cfm. Accessed March 12, 2015.

15. Rosenbloom AH, Jotkowitz A. The ethics of the hospitalist model. J Hosp Med 2010;5(3):183–8.

16. Nelson JR, Whitcomb WF. NAIP position on the voluntary use of inpatient physicians. Hospitalist 1999;3:6–7.

17. Wachter RM. Hospital medicine. 1st edition. Philadelphia: Lippincott Williams and Wilkins; 2000.

18. Glasheen JJ. Hospital medicine secrets. Philadelphia: Elsevier Health Sciences; 2006.

19. Williams M. Comprehensive hospital medicine: an evidence based approach. Philadelphia: Saunders Elsevier; 2007.

20. McKean S. Principles and practice of hospital medicine. New York: McGraw-Hill; 2012.

21. Society of Hospital Medicine. Available at: http://www.hospitalmedicine.org/Web/Education/Core_Competencies.aspx. Accessed February 1, 2015.

22. American Board of Internal Medicine. News. Available at: http://www.abim.org/news/focused-practice-hospital-medicine-questions-answers.aspx. Accessed February 1, 2015.

23. Brown RG. Hospitalist concept: another dangerous trend. Am Fam Physician 1998;58:339–42.

24. Bryant DC. Hospitalists and "officists": preparing for the future of general internal medicine. J Gen Intern Med 1999;14(3):182–5.

25. Stelfox HT, Palmisani S, Scurlock C, et al. The "To Err is Human" report and the patient safety literature. Qual Saf Health Care 2006;15(3):174–8.

26. Brennan T, Leape L, Laird N, et al. Incidence of adverse events and negligence in hospitalized patients: results of the Harvard Medical Practice Study I. 1991. Qual Saf Health Care 2004;13(2):145–52.

27. Whitcomb WF, Nelson JR. President's column. The hospitalist. NAIP. Philadelphia: Spring; 1999.

28. President's address: NAIP Annual Meeting. Philadelphia, PA, April 11–12, 2000.

29. Maynard GA, Budnitz TL, Nickel WK. 2011 John M. Eisenberg Patient Safety and Quality Awards. Mentored implementation: building leaders and achieving results through a collaborative improvement model. Innovation in patient safety and quality at the national level. Jt Comm J Qual Patient Saf 2012;38(7):301–10.

30. Kuo YF, Sharma G, Freeman JL, et al. Growth in the care of older patients by hospitalists in the United States. N Engl J Med 2009;360(11):1102–12.

31. Kralovec PD, Miller JA, Wellikson L, et al. The status of hospital medicine groups in the United States. J Hosp Med 2006;1(2):75–80.

32. Philibert I, Friedmann P, Williams WT. New requirements for resident duty hours. JAMA 2002;288(9):1112–4.

33. Roy CL, Liang CL, Lund M, et al. Implementation of a physician assistant/hospitalist service in an academic medical center: impact on efficiency and patient outcomes. J Hosp Med 2008;3(5):361–8.

34. Healthcare cost and utilization project. Available at: http://www.hcup-us.ahrq.gov/reports/statbriefs/sb183-Hospitalizations-Multiple-Chronic-Conditions-Projections-2014.jsp. Accessed February 1, 2015.

35. Park J, Jones K. Use of hospitalists and office-based primary care physicians' productivity. J Gen Intern Med 2014;30(5):572–81.

36. Nelson JR, Wellikson L, Wachter RM. Specialty hospitalists: analyzing an emerging phenomenon. JAMA 2012;307(16):1699–700.

37. Society of Hospital Medicine. 2014 State of Hospital medicine report. Available at: www.hospitalmedicine.org/survey2014. Accessed February 9, 2015.

38. Hoff TH, Whitcomb WF, Williams K, et al. Characteristics and work experiences of hospitalists in the United States. Arch Intern Med 2001;161:851–8.

39. Huddelston JM, Long KH, Naessens JM, et al, Hospitalist–Orthopedic Team Trial Investigators. Medical and surgical comanagement after elective hip and knee arthroplasty: a randomized, controlled trial. Ann Intern Med 2004;141(1):28–38.

40. Pantilat SZ. End-of-life care for the hospitalized patient. Med Clin North Am 2002;86:749–70.

41. Wachter RM, Katz P, Showstack J, et al. Reorganizing an academic medical service: impact on cost, quality, patient satisfaction, and education. JAMA 1998;279:1560–5.

42. Meltzer D, Manning WG, Morrison J, et al. Effects of physician experience on costs and outcomes on an academic general medicine service: results of a trial of hospitalists. Ann Intern Med 2002;137(11):866–74.

43. Coffman J, Rundall TG. The impact of hospitalists on the cost and quality of inpatient care in the United States: a research synthesis. Med Care Res Rev 2005;62(4):379–406.

44. Lindenauer PK, Rothberg MB, Pekow PS, et al. Outcomes of care by hospitalists, general internists, and family physicians. N Engl J Med 2007;357(25):2589–600.

45. Jungerwirth R, Wheeler SB, Paul JE. Association of hospitalist presence and hospital-level outcome measures among Medicare patients. J Hosp Med 2014;9(1):1–6.

46. Dall L, Simmons T, Peterson S, et al. Beta-blocker use in patients with acute myocardial infarction treated by hospitalists. Manag Care Interface 2000;13(5):61–3.

47. Roytman MM, Thomas SM, Jiang CS. Comparison of practice patterns of hospitalists and community physicians in the care of patients with congestive heart failure. J Hosp Med 2008;3(1):35–41.

48. Lindenauer PK, Chehabeddine R, Pekow P, et al. Quality of care for patients hospitalized with heart failure: assessing the impact of hospitalists. Arch Intern Med 2002;162(11):1251–6.

49. Chen LM, Birkmeyer JD, Saint S, et al. Hospitalist staffing and patient satisfaction in the national Medicare population. J Hosp Med 2013;8(3):126–31.

50. White HL, Glazier RH. Do hospitalist physicians improve the quality of inpatient care delivery? A systematic review of process, efficiency and outcome measures. BMC Med 2011;9:58.

51. Kuo YF, Goodwin JS. Association of hospitalist care with medical utilization after discharge: evidence of cost shift from a cohort study. Ann Intern Med 2011;155(3):152–9.

52. Turner J, Hansen L, Hinami K, et al. The impact of hospitalist discontinuity on hospital cost, readmissions, and patient satisfaction. J Gen Intern Med 2014;29(7):1004–8.

53. Goodrich K, Krumholz HM, Conway PH, et al. Hospitalist utilization and hospital performance on 6 publicly reported patient outcomes. J Hosp Med 2012;7(6): 482–8.
54. Available at: www.hospitalmedicine.org/resourcerooms. Accessed February 1, 2015.
55. Hansen LO, Greenwald JL, Budnitz T, et al. Project BOOST: Effectiveness of a multihospital effort to reduce rehospitalization. J Hosp Med 2013;8:421–7.
56. Wachter RM. Hospitalists in the United States: mission accomplished or work-in-progress. N Engl J Med 2004;350:1935–6.
57. Roberts DL, Cannon KJ, Wellik KE, et al. Burnout in inpatient-based versus outpatient-based physicians: a systematic review and meta-analysis. J Hosp Med 2013;8(11):653–64.
58. Hinami K, Whelan CT, Miller JA, et al. Person-job fit: an exploratory cross-sectional analysis of hospitalists. J Hosp Med 2013;8(2):96–101.
59. Elliott DJ, Young RS, Brice J, et al. Effect of hospitalist workload on the quality and efficiency of care. JAMA Intern Med 2014;174(5):786–93.
60. The American Congress of Obstetricians and Gynecologists. Available at: http://www.acog.org/About-ACOG/ACOG-Departments/Practice-Management-and-Managed-Care/The-Laborist—A-Flexible-Concept. Accessed February 9, 2015.
61. Cowan MJ, Shapiro M, Hays RD, et al. The effect of a multidisciplinary hospitalist/physician and advanced practice nurse collaboration on hospital costs. J Nurs Adm 2006;36(2):79–85.
62. Meltzer DO, Ruhnke GW. Redesigning care for patients at increased hospitalization risk: the Comprehensive Care Physician model. Health Aff (Millwood) 2014; 33(5):770–7.
63. Doctoroff L, Nijhawan A, McNally D, et al. The characteristics and impact of a hospitalist-staffed post-discharge clinic. Am J Med 2013;126(11):1016.e9–15.
64. Burke RE, Whitfield E, Prochazka AV. Effect of a hospitalist-run postdischarge clinic on outcomes. J Hosp Med 2014;9(1):7–12.
65. Singh S, Fletcher KE. A qualitative evaluation of geographical localization of hospitalists: how unintended consequences may impact quality. J Gen Intern Med 2014;29(7):1009–16.
66. O'Leary KJ, Haviley C, Slade ME, et al. Improving teamwork: impact of structured interdisciplinary rounds on a hospitalist unit. J Hosp Med 2011;6(2):88–93.
67. Stein J, Payne C, Methvin A, et al. Reorganizing a hospital ward as an accountable care unit. J Hosp Med 2015;10(1):36–40.
68. Kim CS, King E, Stein J, et al. Unit-based interprofessional leadership models in six US hospitals. J Hosp Med 2014;9(8):545–50.
69. Olson R, Garite TJ, Fishman A, et al. Obstetrician/gynecologist hospitalists: can we improve safety and outcomes for patients and hospitals and improve lifestyle for physicians? Am J Obstet Gynecol 2012;207(2):81–6.

Hospitalists and Their Impact on Quality, Patient Safety, and Satisfaction

Flora Kisuule, MD, MPH, Eric E. Howell, MD*

KEYWORDS

- Generalist hospitalist • Patient safety • Quality improvement • Patient satisfaction
- Obstetric-gynecologic hospitalist

KEY POINTS

- Hospitalists are playing key roles in patient safety, quality improvement, and patient satisfaction as either leaders or practitioners in the field.
- Primary care specialties formed the basis of hospitalist programs; however, several subspecialties are now involved in hospitalist programs.
- Like other specialty hospitalists, the obstetric-gynecologist (OB/Gyn) hospitalist model emerged out of the broader need for improved patient safety and provision of quality care.

BACKGROUND

Since the initial description of hospitalists by Wachter and Goldman[1] in 1996, hospitalist roles have evolved in breadth and sophistication. Hospitalists have proved to be adept as clinicians, teachers, safety and quality officers, and executives in the C-suite. The hospitalist field emerged as a response to a combination of forces, including primary care providers providing less inpatient care, the need for 24/7 on-site high-value patient care, changes in Accreditation Council for Graduate Medical Education (ACGME) regulations, comanagement opportunities, and hospitalists being selected for leadership roles.[2]

During the 1990s, the initial years of the hospitalist movement, growth in the field was driven largely by clinical coverage needs and improving efficiency. Reducing both length of stay and cost, while maintaining or improving outcomes, was a major benefit of early hospitalist programs.[3] At that time, there were no external forces

Disclosure: Nothing to report.
Division of Hospital Medicine, Department of Medicine, Johns Hopkins Bayview Medical Center, Johns Hopkins University School of Medicine, 5200 Eastern Avenue, MFL West, 6th Floor, Baltimore, MD 21224, USA
* Corresponding author.
E-mail address: ehowell@jhmi.edu

Obstet Gynecol Clin N Am 42 (2015) 433–446
http://dx.doi.org/10.1016/j.ogc.2015.05.003
0889-8545/15/$ – see front matter © 2015 Elsevier Inc. All rights reserved.

obgyn.theclinics.com

promoting patient safety and quality. Then, in 1999, the Institute of Medicine (IOM) launched the patient safety movement when it published the report "To Err is Human."[4] The report estimated that up to 98,000 patients died annually because of medical errors and caused a paradigm shift on how the public viewed health care. According to the IOM report, the hospital was a dangerous place, a message that resonated with numerous hospitalists who began to engage in patient safety efforts as part of their careers. This IOM message received widespread attention in the lay press, engaged providers of all types, and led to progress in patient safety efforts. The patient safety movement continued to gain momentum in the early 2000s, with efforts to enforce safety standards through regulation, complete with consequences for nonadherence.[5] The Joint Commission developed a process to introduce new safety standards that included engaging patients and their caregivers in the development. The Joint Commission also started unannounced visits to hospitals, and for the first time in history, hospital accreditation was no longer guaranteed.[5] Hospitalists have been a critical partner in the patient safety movement, often driving change from the front lines as clinicians, as leaders in the C-suite, and even within the Centers for Medicare and Medicaid Services (CMS) itself.

Quality improvement initiatives for systems of care are now critical for any hospital. Until recently, a hospital's financial performance was based solely on transactions, and was not linked to quality or other performance outcomes. Within the past 5 years CMS began using financial incentives in an effort to reward for quality, a first for that organization. In 2010, Wachter[5] wrote, "by 2015, a hospital's Medicare reimbursement will be at risk through a variety of initiatives including value based purchasing and meaningful use standards...private payers are replicating Medicare's standards, particularly when they perceive that they may lead to both improved quality and lower costs." These predictions are indeed reality. Hospitals now receive a publically available scorecard for quality and safety through CMS (hospitalcompare.gov) with financial outcomes linked to specific metrics. In total, at least 5.5% of Medicare dollars are linked to quality measures in 2015, including mortality, readmission rates, patient-centered care, and other clinical outcomes.

The IOM followed up on its 1999 report by publishing *Crossing the Quality Chasm* in 2001; it outlined patient-centered care as 1 of their 6 aims necessary to improve the health care delivery system.[6] The premise was that patients who are involved in their treatment plan are more likely to be satisfied with their overall hospital experience and have better outcomes.[7] Patient-centered care is now also in the public opinion arena. The Agency for Healthcare Research and Quality (AHRQ) developed the Hospital Consumer Assessment of Healthcare Providers and Systems (HCAHPS) survey. This survey was designed to assess hospitalized patients' experience with care.[8] The results are publicly reported by CMS and, as previously mentioned, also affect hospital reimbursement.

Many of the forces that drove the growth of generalist hospitalists over the past 15 to 20 years also apply to specialty hospitalists, including OB/Gyn hospitalists. Generalist hospitalists have been successful in the venues of patient safety, quality, and patient-centered care. A closer look at the work by generalist hospitalists in these areas can provide guidance to specialty hospitalists as they work to affect the provision of care for their patients.

HOSPITALISTS AND PATIENT SAFETY

Despite the emphasis on improving patient safety over the past 15 years, high rates of medical injury continue to persist. Some studies show that 1 in 3 hospitalized patients still suffer preventable harm.[9] As they have since the 1999 IOM report, hospitalists continue to play key roles in patient safety and quality improvement, either as leaders or as practitioners in the field. There are several areas in the literature in which generalist hospitalists are deeply involved and take the lead to improve patient safety. Specific examples are as follows:

- Efforts to understand and reduce device-associated morbidity and mortality
- Improving medication safety
- Venous thromboembolism (VTE) prophylaxis

Device-Associated Morbidity

Several devices are associated with increased morbidity in the hospital setting. Examples include urinary catheters, central or peripheral lines, and ventilators. Deep vein thrombosis (DVT) and bloodstream infections are well-known risks associated with peripherally inserted central catheters (PICCs).[10] Other complications associated with PICCs include superficial thrombophlebitis and mechanical complications. Hospitalists play a major role in making the decision to insert and manage these catheters. Aside from the morbidity associated with the presence of the devices themselves, there is a potential for harm stemming from variability in practices of hospitalists when making the decision to place and maintain these lines. As an example of hospitalists improving patient safety related to PICCs, one hospitalist group led a patient safety program to define the scope of the work needed to improve practice related to these devices.[10] Specific areas of concern that they identified in the use of PICCs are as follows:

- Forgetting that a patient has a PICC
- Inserting a PICC in a patient who simultaneously has a peripheral line
- Placing a line that is avoidable
- Variations in treatment duration for PICC-associated DVT.

The identification of areas of concern related to devices allows for targeted interventions to be developed to mitigate the impact to patient safety.

Medication Safety

Approximately one-third of hospitalized patients are adults aged 65 years and older.[11] One unique challenge posed by this patient population is that about half take at least 5 medications daily. Polypharmacy adds a level of complexity when making treatment decisions and often necessitates medication changes when the patient is hospitalized. Harris and colleagues[11] performed a study to characterize changes in medication regimens made during a hospitalization and evaluated postdischarge medication adherence. The investigators found medication changes because of home medications being stopped during the hospitalization. Additional medication changes were due to unintentional errors of omission, such as previous home medications not being listed on discharge paperwork. These errors occurred because medications were not appropriately captured at the time of admission and were therefore not given to the patient at any point during their hospitalization, including discharge. Of the home medications that were appropriately documented and then continued, there were often changes in dosing frequency or strength. Finally, in addition to changes to existing home medications, approximately 2 new medications were prescribed for each discharged older adult. A 3-day postdischarge follow-up phone call showed medication compliance rates ranging from 75% to 90%. Although adherence was high, the patients did not follow all recommendations regarding their medications at discharge.

Coleman and colleagues[12] also performed a study aimed at quantifying the prevalence and contributing factors leading to posthospital medication discrepancies. The investigators found that 14% of patients experienced one or more medication discrepancies. The contributing factors were evenly split between patients themselves and the health care system. About 14% of the patients who had medication discrepancies were readmitted when compared with 6% of the patients who did not have medication discrepancies. This difference was statistically significant.

Medication safety remains an area in need of continued intervention. The literature identifies several areas in which hospitalists have articulated the problems, highlighted the magnitude of the problem, and identified key determinants of the problem. As a specialty, hospital medicine has recognized that more work needs to be done to identify and implement solutions to the patient safety issues surrounding medications.

Venous Thromboembolism Prophylaxis

VTE is a common cause of morbidity and mortality in hospitalized patients, and more patients die each year from VTE than do from motor vehicle accidents.[13] Research by hospitalists in this area has shown that rates of pharmacologic prophylaxis are low in US hospitals.[14] The Joint Commission and the CMS has a performance measure for VTE prophylaxis aimed at increasing the rate of prophylaxis in hospitalized patients. The Society of Hospital Medicine (SHM) has supported hospitalists in their endeavors toward system-based initiatives to improve quality of care. The VTE quality improvement room was the first practice-based resource developed by SHM and has been widely successful in engaging multiple hospitals and hospitalists in improving VTE outcomes.[15]

HOSPITALISTS AND QUALITY

Quality improvement remains a priority for virtually all hospitals around the country. Hospitalists call hospitals home and are well positioned to lead the efforts in this area. Early in the development of hospitalists as quality champions, it was recognized that there are facilitators and barriers to completing patient safety and quality improvement initiatives (**Box 1**).[16] To the credit of the specialty as a whole, many of these barriers have been addressed on both the local and national scale. Hospitalists have had the support of a national organization, the SHM, to help develop skills and resources important to leading change. In addition, local hospitalists have been willing to grow as leaders advocating for change and participating in complex organizational initiatives. A closer look at the work of generalist hospitalists can lay a blueprint for work that could be done by OB/Gyn hospitalists in the area of quality. Specific examples are

- Care transitions
- Comanagement
- Palliative care

Care Transitions

Care transitions are a period of high risk for patients. At every transition, there is a risk of missed or inaccurate information relayed, duplication of testing, and medication discrepancies. Care transitions at the time of admission and hospital discharge are common, as are transitions between hospitalists who are rotating on and off service. There has been much focus given to the transition during the hospital discharge

---

Box 1
Facilitators and barriers to patient safety initiatives

Facilitators of patient safety initiatives

- Having a champion or process owner
- Having resources for project management and data collection
- Having a multidisciplinary effort
- Having leadership backing
- Using established QI methodology

Barriers to patient safety initiatives

- New process avoidance
- Inertia
- Patient variability
- Having no process owner or champion

---

because approximately 20% of Medicare beneficiaries are readmitted within 30 days (**Fig. 1**) and there is wide variation between regions.[17] In addition, as of October 2012, hospitals incur financial penalties for excess readmissions. Hospitals nationwide have developed initiatives aimed at improving readmission rates. Drill downs of the root causes surrounding readmissions point at inadequate care coordination during transitions of care. Optimizing care coordination efforts and improved handoffs are critical as patient complexity and care fragmentation increases. The AHRQ defines care coordination as "deliberately organizing patient care activities and sharing information among all the participants concerned with a patient's care to achieve safer and more effective care."[18] Challenges to care coordination include lack of time, inability to reach providers by phone, lack of personal relationships with clinicians in a different setting, medication list discrepancies, and difficulties obtaining follow-up appointments.

Hospitalists are in the forefront of efforts to improve care coordination. The SHM developed the project Better Outcomes by Optimizing Safe Transitions (BOOST) with the aim of improving discharge transitions from hospital to home. Project BOOST has several overarching goals and has focused on key aspects of the hospital discharge transition (**Box 2**).[19] Project BOOST provides individualized physician mentoring, which has helped with the implementation of BOOST interventions at more than 100 hospitals.

On a smaller scale, hospitalists have engaged in site-specific interventions with some success at improving care coordination. For example, Dedhia and colleagues[20] developed a tool kit to improve the transition of older adults from the hospital to their homes. This tool kit had the following 5 core elements: admission form with geriatric cues, fax to the primary care provider notifying them of the admission, interdisciplinary work sheet to identify barriers to discharge, pharmacist-physician collaborative medication reconciliation, and predischarge planning appointments. This hospitalist-driven initiative on the hospitalist service of 3 hospitals showed that a multidisciplinary and multifaceted effort can positively affect the care of older adults in their transition from the hospital to home.

Another area of great concern is transitioning patients from the emergency department (ED) into an inpatient bed. The IOM considers the current state of EDs in crisis

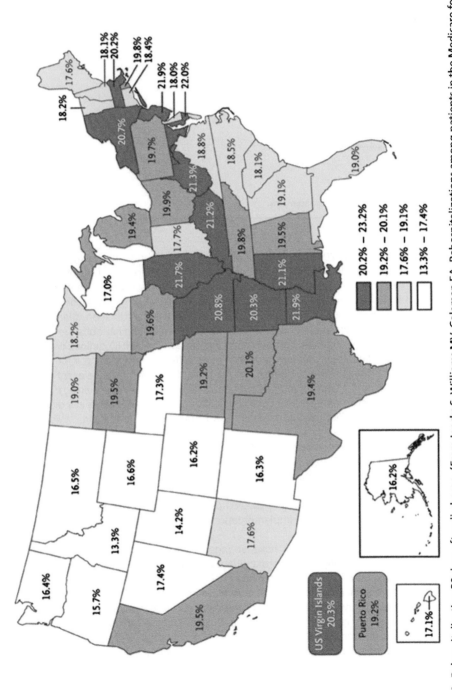

Fig. 1. Rehospitalization 30 days after discharge. (*From* Jencks S, Williams MV, Coleman EA. Rehospitalizations among patients in the Medicare fee-for-service program. N Engl J Med 2009;360:1424; with permission.)

> **Box 2**
> **Project BOOST: goals and key aspects**
>
> Goals
>
> - Assist hospitals in improving their patients' discharge transition
> - Reduce hospitals' 30-day readmission
> - Improve patient satisfaction
> - Reduce errors in the postdischarge period
>
> Key aspects of hospital discharge transition
>
> - Identification of high-risk patients
> - Preparing patients and their families for discharge
> - Medication reconciliation
> - Improving inpatient and outpatient provider communication
> - Ensuring adequate follow-up and providing technical support

because 91% of them are crowded.[21] Ambulance diversion increases death by 1% per 6 miles driven.[22] ED boarding is associated with poor outcomes such as increased time to antibiotics, increased intensive care unit (ICU) mortality, and increased ICU length of stay.[23] Howell and colleagues[24] worked to improve ED throughput by increasing efficiency of existing physical inpatient space, which they did by instituting active bed management (ABM). The process of ABM involves appointing a triage hospitalist who triages patients from the ED to the entire department of medicine and proactively manages ICU beds. ABM reduced ambulance diversion by 27%.

Comanagement of Surgical Patients

Patients undergoing surgery are increasing in age and number of comorbidities.[25] In addition, simpler surgical procedures have shifted to the outpatient arena leaving sicker, older, and more complex patients in the hospital surgical units.[25] Work duty hours imposed by the ACGME have reduced the ability of surgical residents to respond to patients outside the operating room. Anecdotally, the reduced exposure to medically complex patients outside of the operating room has led to surgical residents who are less comfortable managing these patients' nonsurgical comorbidities. In addition, forces around reimbursement that are not favorable for long length of stay have resulted in the development of comanagement models of surgical patients by hospitalists. Comanagement of surgical patients refers to hospitalists daily assessing and addressing medical problems of hospitalized patients, communicating with surgeons, and facilitating the transition of patients from the hospital.[25] Comanagement by hospitalist has been shown to reduce postoperative medical complications, mortality, rehospitalization, and increase use of evidence-based treatment.[26] Comanagement has also been shown to reduce time to surgery,[27] reduction in ICU admissions,[28] and hospital costs per patient.[28]

The success of the comanagement of surgical patients' model is leading to expansion into the subspecialist arena. In 2014, Desai and colleagues[29] described a model in which comanagement between a hospitalist and hepatologist improved the quality of care of inpatients with chronic liver disease. When comparing this model with a conventional model that involved just hepatologists, the comanagement model resulted in a greater proportion of patients undergoing paracentesis within 24 hours, more frequent and appropriate avoidance of fresh frozen plasma use, a greater percentage of patients with appropriate reception of albumin, and more patients discharged on spontaneous bacterial peritonitis prophylaxis. The investigators also noted a trend in improved outcomes related to ICU transfer, inpatient mortality, 30-day readmission, and mortality rates.

End-of-Life/Palliative Care

Palliative care has been identified by the SHM as a core competency in hospital medicine. The role of the hospitalist in this field ranges from direct patient care to advocacy for critically ill patients.[30] Specific areas that hospitalists have focused in filling knowledge gaps to improve their provision of end-of-life care are pain and symptom management, understanding hospice eligibility, and communicating bad news.[30] The threats to patient safety surrounding end-of-life care can be failure to follow advanced directives and failure to treat symptoms adequately. An example of work by hospitalists in this area is by Gomutbutra and colleagues[31] who showed that adding benzodiazepines to opioids was associated with improvement in moderate to severe dyspnea in hospitalized patients receiving palliative care. Hospitalists are well positioned to identify these threats to patient safety during end of life and have engaged in identifying solutions so as to bring about the changes necessary to provide safe and effective care to critically ill patients.

HOSPITALISTS AND PATIENT-CENTERED CARE

The IOM defines patient-centered care as "Providing care that is respectful of and responsive to individual patient preferences, needs, and values, and ensuring that patient values guide all clinical decisions."[6] One of the measures for patient-centered care is patient satisfaction. These scores are currently obtained through the HCAHPS survey. While patient-centered care is widely accepted as critical to the practice of medicine, there remains concern among generalist hospitalists on the validity of the HCAHPS measures. One major concern is that multiple providers may be engaged in the care of a patient during a hospitalization, and therefore, attributing the HCAHPS measure to one hospitalist can be problematic. Torok and colleagues[32] developed and validated tool to assess inpatient satisfaction with care from hospitalists (TAISCH). The investigators addressed the following concerns related to current patient satisfaction surveys:

- Several hospitalists and consultants may be involved in the care of one patient
- Only a few questions are asked about a doctors' performance
- The surveys are mailed after discharge with no way to facilitate recall
- Low response rates

TAISCH was built on the quality of care measures that are endorsed by the SHM, which recommends assessing patient satisfaction across 6 domains: physician availability, physician concern for patients, physician communication skills, physician courteousness, physician clinical sills, and physician involvement in patient families. To ensure that patients had true perspective on their doctors, they were only asked to assess physicians who had cared for them for at least 2 consecutive days. The survey was administered while patients were still in the hospital and only if patients could correctly identify their provider. Unlike HCAHPS and Press Ganey, TAISCH provides patient satisfaction data that are timely, have a high response rate, and that can be attributed to specific hospitalists.[32]

EMERGENCE OF SUBSPECIALTY HOSPITALISTS

Generalist training formed the basis of most hospitalist programs during the initial 15 years of the specialty; however, today, several subspecialties are involved in hospitalist programs around the country (**Fig. 2**) (Mr Ethan Gray, Vice President of Membership, Society of Hospital Medicine, personal communication, 2015). Like the initial hospitalist movement, the factors driving the rapid growth of subspecialty hospitalists include

- Nationally mandated quality and safety measures
- Increasing age and complexity of the hospitalized patient
- Reduced residency duty hours
- Increased economic pressures to contain costs and reduce length of stay
- Specialty physicians relinquishing hospital privileges to focus on outpatient practices

The roles of the subspecialty hospitalist are varied. For example, the expertise of the neurohospitalist has broadly been defined as "providing all aspects of neurologic care to both hospitalized and emergency room patients...ultimately neurohospitalists need to provide on-site availability and participate in, if not spearhead, system improvements in quality, efficiency, and safety."[33]

Pediatric hospitalist groups have also exploded in response to public and payer demand for cost-effective high-quality care.[34] Pediatric hospitalist groups have taken on the challenge of improving quality of care by offering services such as palliative care and consults and are serving as the leaders for quality improvement and patient safety in hospitals.[35]

Like other specialty hospitalists, the OB/Gyn hospitalist model emerged out of the broader need for improved patient safety, specifically the realization that bad outcomes result from the lack of immediate availability of a physician in the labor and

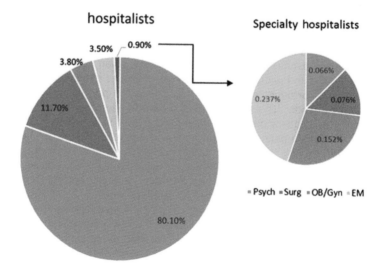

Fig. 2. SHM membership by reported specialty, total n = 10,532. EM, emergency medicine; Psych, psychiatry; Surg, surgery. (*From* Mr Ethan Gray, Vice President of Membership, Society of Hospital Medicine, personal communication, 2015; with permission.)

delivery suite. Other contributing factors were desire among providers to separate hospital-based duties from outpatient for better work-life balance, appeal for shift work as opposed to running a busy private practice, reduced training in critical skills needed during labor and delivery, outpatient focus of obstetrics and gynecology medicine resulting in a void in the care of the laboring patient, and the need for physicians to implement protocols and policies in the hospital.[36] The American College of Obstetrics and Gynecology Committee on Patient safety and Quality has previously stated that it "supports the continued development of the OB/Gyn hospitalist model as one potential approach to achieving increased professional and patient satisfaction while maintaining safe and effective care across delivery settings."[37]

SPECULATION OF IMPACT ON OBSTETRIC-GYNECOLOGIST HOSPITALIST

The forces that led to the rise of the generalist and subspecialty hospitalist movements can be narrowed down to reducing cost and improving the quality of care and safety of the hospitalized patient. Before the OB/Gyn hospitalist, several physicians cared for a few laboring patients at one time, which resulted in handoffs and issues of communication between the labor and delivery nurse and the obstetrician who could be off-site when a patient was in labor.[37] Now, there is an ever-present, OB/GYN hospitalist immediately on-site for any patient. It follows that this improved physician access may lead to fewer medical errors and improve patient safety.

Like their generalist counterparts, OB/Gyn hospitalists use devices in clinical practice, such as uterine tamponade balloons. The presence of these hospitalists in hospitals means that they are readily available for in-servicing as well as for authoring and implementing hospital-based policies to ensure patient safety and reduce device-associated morbidity. Olson and colleagues[36] describe a scenario in which a new uterine tamponade balloon device was introduced at a hospital and several training sessions were offered to all obstetric department physicians. Relatively few nonhospitalist physicians attended, whereas all the OB/Gyn hospitalists did. The OB/Gyn hospitalists went on to become device experts and placed more of the balloons than all nonhospitalist obstetricians combined.

OB/Gyn hospitalists have to hand over care, when they complete a shift as well as transfer care to the outpatient OB/Gyn physician as patient's leave the hospitals. The challenges surrounding coordination of care are important areas for the OB/Gyn hospitalist to ponder. These providers also have to develop procedures and protocols to ensure that patient care is seamless, safe, and satisfactory. In addition, while the typical OB/Gyn patient may not be as advanced in age as the typical hospitalized medicine patient, the OB/Gyn hospitalist will likely also experience older women in the labor and delivery suite. More women are having their children at an older age[38] because they take out time to plan and develop their careers. This fact may result in patients with more comorbidities or at higher risks of complications. Special processes such as comanagement might need to be developed by OB/Gyn hospitalists to ensure patient safety and satisfaction. Furthermore, as the population ages, OB/Gyn hospitalists may find themselves managing nonobstetric illnesses in the hospital setting. These patients will have the same challenges as their medicine counterparts such as polypharmacy and the potential for medication errors. OB/Gyn hospitalists will need to develop protocols to ensure medication safety when these patients are discharged. VTE prophylaxis is already an area of focus in OB/Gyn, and refining the care of patients in this area is important. Finally, while the concept of palliative care seems incongruent with the specialty of OB/Gyn, the laboring patient can have adverse outcomes too. Neonates and babies have the highest death rates in the pediatric population.[39] Still births and having a child after a still birth require some of the same end-of-life skills such as giving bad news and helping a patient with grief and loss. Perinatal palliative care is a developing specialty, and OB/Gyn hospitalists could fill some of these roles.

As OB/Gyn hospitalists settle into their role, they will begin to assume leadership in ensuring that quality improvement initiatives specific to their practice are met. These hospitalists will begin to design interventions and plan initiatives to ensure patient safety. Finally, they will have to work to provide patient-centered care and will be measured on this, in part, by how satisfied the patients are with the care they receive. As society continues to demand patient-centered care, it will be important to ensure that patients are satisfied with the services that they receive from their hospitals and from their providers. The way patient satisfaction is currently measured has significant limitations. Generalist hospitalists are once again leading the way in improving this process by developing tools such as TAISCH that more accurately measure patients' satisfaction with their hospitalist providers. Measuring patient satisfaction in a more accurate way is going to become important for OB/Gyn hospitalists so that they can give meaningful, targeted feedback that will motivate individual providers to improve their practice. Furthermore, conscientious management of hospital beds by hospitalists providing ABM has had a positive and substantial impact on the ED throughput of critically ill patients admitted to ICU beds. This efficiency is likely to have affected patient satisfaction and safety. The OB/Gyn hospitalist could develop similar roles to ensure speedy throughput of laboring mothers through labor and delivery suites.

SUMMARY

Since the hospitalist concept was introduced nearly 20 years ago, hospitalists have shown numerous advantages, namely, 24/7 availability, greater familiarity with hospital systems, improved cost, and providing leadership in the areas of quality improvement, patient safety, and patient satisfaction. OB/Gyn hospitalists are showing similar successes as their generalist counterparts by being readily available to the laboring patients. As the field grows, the OB/Gyn hospitalist will need to determine the skill set necessary to be considered an OB/Gyn hospitalist. A defining moment in the general internal medicine hospitalist movement was the development and publishing of the core competencies in hospital medicine. These competencies standardize the skill set expected of a practicing hospitalist. The competencies are divided into 3 sections: clinical conditions, procedures, and health care systems.[40] Quality improvement and patient safety are listed in the section on health care systems.[40] Every practicing hospitalist (generalist and specialist) should expect to affect the care of their patient in these areas. The pediatric hospitalists have also developed and published their core competencies in pediatric hospital medicine; they have divided their competencies into 4 sections: common clinical diagnoses and conditions, core skills, specialized clinical services, and health care systems.[41] These hospitalists also list continuous quality improvement and patient safety as a core competency for their field. As the field of OB/Gyn hospital medicine grows, it will be important to define core competencies to guide curriculum development and provide direction for the field. Like their generalist counterparts, the areas of quality improvement and patient safety will need to be important components of the competencies if the field is to continue to thrive.

The SHM provides resources for programs to build quality and safety initiatives at hospitalists' home institutions. The partnership between the newly developed Society of OB/GYN Hospitalists (formed in 2011), and the SHM holds promise for OB/GYN hospitalists in defining their professional agenda and in improving quality and safety in the practice of hospital-based obstetric patient care.

The success of the internal medicine hospitalist movement has resulted in the growth and expansion of specialty hospitalists. OB/Gyn hospitalists have sprouted out of the same need. In their roles, they are poised to provide the same benefits as their internal medicine counterparts.

REFERENCES

1. Wachter RM, Goldman L. The emerging role of the "hospitalists" in the American Health Care System. N Engl J Med 1996;335(7):514–7.
2. Wachter RM. The hospitalist field turns 15: new opportunities and challenges. J Hosp Med 2011;6(4):E1–4.
3. Wachter RM, Goldman L. The hospitalist movement 5 years later. JAMA 2002; 287(4):487–94.
4. Corrigan J, Kohn L, Donaldson M, editors. To err is human: building a safer health system. Washington, DC: National Academy Press; Institute of Medicine; 1999.
5. Wachter RM. Patient safety at ten: unmistakable progress, troubling gaps. Health Aff 2010;29:165–73.
6. Committee on Quality of Health Care in America, Institute of Medicine. Crossing the quality chasm: a new health system for the 21st century. Washington, DC: National Academy Press; 2001.
7. Farberg AS, Lin AM, Kuhn L, et al. Dear doctor: a tool to facilitate patient-centered communication. J Hosp Med 2013;8(10):553–8.
8. O'Leary KH, Afsar-Manest N, Budnitz T, et al. Hospital quality and patient safety competencies: development, description, and recommendations for use. J Hosp Med 2011;6(9):530–6.
9. Pronovost PJ, Miller MR, Wachter RM. Tracking progress in patient safety: an elusive target. JAMA 2006;296(6):696–9.
10. Chopra V, Kuhn L, Krien S, et al. Hospitalist experiences, practice, opinions, and knowledge regarding peripherally inserted central catheters: results of a National Survey. J Hosp Med 2013;8(11):635–8.
11. Harris CM, Sridharan A, Wright S, et al. What happens to the medication regimens of older adults during and after an acute hospitalization. J Patient Saf 2013;9(3):150–3.
12. Coleman EA, Smith JD, Raha D. Posthospital medication discrepancies. Arch Intern Med 2005;165:1842–7.
13. Venous Thromboembolism (VTE) Prevention in the Hospital: Transcript. June 2010. Agency for Healthcare Research and Quality, Rockville, MD. Available at: http://archive.ahrq.gov/professionals/quality-patient-safety/quality-resources/value/vtepresentation/maynardtranscr.html. Accessed December 15, 2014.
14. Flanders SA, Green T, Bernstein SJ, et al. Hospital performance for pharmacologic venous thromboembolism prophylaxis and rate of venous thromboembolism: a cohort study. JAMA 2014;147(10):1577–84.
15. Stein J, Maynard G. Preventing hospital-acquired venous thromboembolism, a guide for effective quality improvement, version 3.3. Society of Hospital Medicine website, Venous Thromboembolism Quality Implementation Tool Kit. Available at: http://www.hospitalmedicine.org. Accessed December 15, 2014.
16. Flanders SA, Kaufman SR, Parekh VI. Hospitalists as emerging leaders in patient safety: lessons learned and future directions. J Patient Saf 2009;5(1):3–8.

17. Jencks S, Williams MV, Coleman EA. Rehospitalization among patients in the Medicare fee-for-service program. N Engl J Med 2009;360:1418–28.
18. Jones CD, Maihan VB, Dewalt DA, et al. A Failure to communicate: a qualitative exploration of care coordination between hospitals and primary care providers around patient hospitalizations. J Gen Intern Med 2015;30:417–24.
19. Hansen L, Greenwald J, Williams M, et al. Project BOOST: effectiveness of a multihospital effort to reduce rehospitalization. J Hosp Med 2013;8(8): 421–7.
20. Dedhia P, Kravet S, Howell E, et al. A quality improvement intervention to facilitate the transition of older adults from three hospitals back to their homes. J Am Geriatr Soc 2009;57:1540–6.
21. Committee on the Future of Emergency Care in the United States, Institute of Medicine. Hospital-based emergency care: at the breaking point. Washington, DC: National Academics Press; 2007.
22. Nicholl J, West J, Goodacre S, et al. The relationship between distance to hospital and patient mortality in emergencies: an observational study. Emerg Med J 2007; 24(9):665–8.
23. Burt CW, McCaig LF, Valverde RH. Analysis of ambulance transports and diversions among US emergency departments. Ann Emerg Med 2006;47(4):317–26.
24. Howell EE, Bessman E, Marshal R, et al. Hospitalist bed management effecting throughput from the emergency department to the intensive care unit. J Crit Care 2010;25(2):184–9.
25. Huang J. Co-management of surgical patients. J Med Pract Manage 2014;29(6): 348–50.
26. Fisher AA, Davis MW, Rubenach SE, et al. Outcomes for older patients with hip fractures: the impact of orthopedic and geriatric medicine cocare. J Orthop Trauma 2006;20:172–80.
27. Phy MP, Vanness DJ, Melton LJ, et al. Effects of a hospitalist model on elderly patients with hip fracture. Arch Intern Med 2005;165:796–801.
28. Della Rocca G, Moylan KC, Crist BD, et al. Comanagement of geriatric patients with hip fractures: a retrospective, controlled, cohort study. Geriatr Orthop Surg Rehabil 2013;4:10–5.
29. Desai AP, Satoskar R, Appannagari A, et al. Co-management between hospitalist and hepatologist improves the quality of care of inpatients with chronic liver disease. J Clin Gastroenterol 2014;48:e30–6.
30. Kutner JS. Ensuring safe, quality care for hospitalized people with advanced illness, a core obligation for hospitalists. J Hosp Med 2001;2(6):355–6.
31. Gomutbutra P, O'Rirdan DL, Pantilat SZ. Management of moderate-to-severe dyspnea in hospitalized patients receiving palliative care. J Pain Symptom Manage 2013;45(5):885–91.
32. Torok H, Ghazarian S, Kotwal S. Development and validation of the tool to assess inpatient satisfaction with care from hospitalists. J Hosp Med 2014;9:553–8.
33. Chang I, Pratt P. Neurohospitalists: an emerging subspecialty. Curr Neurol Neurosci Rep 2012;12:481–8.
34. Freed LG, Dunham KM. Pediatric hospitalists: training, current practice, and career goals. J Hosp Med 2009;4:179–86.
35. Teufel RJ, Garber M, Taylor RC. Pediatric hospitalist: a national and regional trend. J S C Med Assoc 2007;103(5):126–9.
36. Olson R, Garite TJ, Andreas IF, et al. Obstetrician/gynecologist hospitalists: can we improve safety and outcomes for patients and hospitals and improve lifestyle for physicians. Am J Obstet Gynecol 2012;207(2):81–6.

37. Committee opinion No. 459: The obstetric-gynecologic hospitalist. Obstet Gynecol 2010;116(1):237–9.

38. Mathews TJ, Hamilton BE. Delayed childbearing: more women are having their first child later in life. NCHS Data Brief 2009;21:1–8.

39. Kiman R, Doumic L. Perinatal palliative care: a developing specialty. Int J Palliat Nurs 2014;20(3):143–8.

40. The core competencies in hospital medicine: a framework for faculty development by the society of hospital medicine. J Hosp Med 2006;1(1):2–95.

41. Stucky ER, Maniscalco J, Ottolini MC. Introduction to the pediatric hospital medicine core competencies. J Hosp Med 2010;5:V–VI.

Roles of Obstetrician-Gynecologist Hospitalists with Changes in the Obstetrician-Gynecologist Workforce and Practice

Jennifer A. Tessmer-Tuck, MD[a],*, William F. Rayburn, MD, MBA[b]

KEYWORDS

• Hospitalists • Obstetrician-gynecologists • Workforce • OB-GYN hospitalists
• Laborists

KEY POINTS

- A shortage of OB-GYNs is impending as the adult female population expands, as more uninsured women obtain medical coverage, and as a growing number of OB-GYNs work fewer hours, pursue subspecialties, or retire.
- Changes in the future OB-GYN practice will be more office-based, efficient, and oriented toward standardizing practices and improving the patient experience.
- OB-GYN hospitalist positions offer more of an opportunity to control schedules and work-life balance according to their lifestyle and life-stage needs.
- OB-GYN hospitalists play important roles in standardizing inpatient care and in providing more quality care and performance improvement while attempting to control costs.

INTRODUCTION

Obstetricians-gynecologists (OB-GYNs) represent the fourth largest group of physicians, just behind the traditional primary care fields of internal medicine, family and community medicine, and pediatrics.[1] They represent the only medical specialty dedicated solely to women's health care. Adult women make up approximately two-fifths of the entire US population, with half of those being of reproductive age.[2] The specialty

The authors report no conflict of interest.
[a] Department of Obstetrics and Gynecology, North Memorial Medical Center, Robbinsdale, MN, USA; [b] Department of Obstetrics and Gynecology, The University of New Mexico School of Medicine, Albuquerque, NM, USA
* Corresponding author. 3300 Oakdale Avenue North, Robbinsdale, MN 55422.
E-mail address: Jennifer.tessmertuck@gmail.com

is unique because of its roles in providing 24-7 inpatient obstetrical coverage, surgical services and rapidly evolving ambulatory services incorporating wellness and preventive care.

Like other medical specialties, obstetrics and gynecology has faced a myriad of changes that impact delivery of women's health care. Several of these changes threaten the traditional OB-GYN practice. Despite a steady increase in the US population, the number of OB-GYN resident graduates has expanded negligibly (0.05% per year) to provide the same volume of care.[2] Despite significant increases in the number of US allopathic and osteopathic medical school graduates, the supply of OB-GYNs is not anticipated to increase because of a lack of funding of additional residency positions.

This article identifies and reviews several changes in the OB-GYN workforce and practices. Some will be more unique, and others will be universal to clinical medicine. We then describe how these changes will impact the evolution of the OB-GYN hospitalist movement and its role in the foreseeable future.

CHANGES IN THE OBSTETRICIAN-GYNECOLOGIST WORKFORCE AND PRACTICES
More Female Obstetricians-Gynecologists

More than half of Fellows of the American College of Obstetricians and Gynecologists (ACOG) are women, and more than 80% of OB-GYN residents are women (**Fig. 1**).[2] What impact does this feminization of obstetrics and gynecology have on the workforce? Overall, female physicians work fewer hours and are more likely to work part-time than male physicians. Among OB-GYNs surveyed between 1990 and 2002, women worked fewer hours per week, saw fewer patients per week, took call-duty less frequently, and were less likely to work more than 60 hours per week.[3–6] Not surprisingly, this reduction in work hours correlates with a reduction in

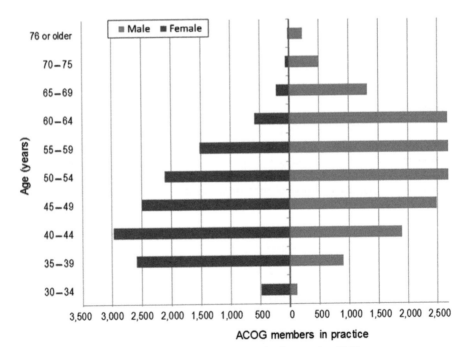

Fig. 1. Age distribution of ACOG members in practice by gender, 2014.

professional productivity. Compared with their male counterparts, female OB-GYNs attend fewer births and perform fewer gynecologic surgeries.[3,6] These gaps in work hours and productivity are more pronounced between male and female OB-GYNs younger than 40.[6]

More contemporary data corroborate these earlier findings. A 2004 national survey found that female OB-GYNs worked significantly fewer hours than male physicians, both weekly and "on-call."[7] Full-time male OB-GYNs nationally older than 50 worked more hours per week than their female counterparts, whereas female OB-GYNs younger than 50 were more likely to work part-time than their male counterparts.[8]

Life stage and, in particular, parenting seems to have a major impact on the hours female physicians work. Married female physicians with children spend more hours per week on parenting and domestic duties than male physicians.[9] Married female OB-GYNs with children worked fewer hours than married male OB-GYNs with children and were more likely to work part-time.

More female OB-GYNs younger than 40 report reducing their hours or stopping practice altogether to meet family or parenting needs, compared with male OB-GYNs in the same age group.[3,10] This may be influenced by partner work status. Although close to 90% of female physician spouses worked full-time, fewer than 45% of male physician spouses worked full-time. Additionally, male physician spouses were 4 times more likely to be employed part-time or not at all.[9] After controlling for other personal and professional factors, conflicts between work and home responsibilities were independently associated with female surgeons reporting a moderate or higher likelihood of planning to reduce their clinical work hours and leave their current practice in the next 24 months.[11,12]

Emphasis on Work-Life Balance

In 1989, Schwartz and colleagues[13] identified that graduating US medical students preferred specialties with a perceived better work-life balance or controllable lifestyles than those with perceived worse work-life balance or uncontrollable lifestyles. Obstetrics and gynecology was ranked among the "noncontrollable" lifestyle specialties. After controlling for income, work hours, and years of graduate medical education required, work with a "controllable lifestyle" explained specialty preference of many female and male medical students.[14] The controllable lifestyle specialties were appealing to both female and male students, and almost doubled in popularity between 1996 and 2003.[15,16]

In 2008, 91% of female American Medical Association members identified "achieving work-life balance" as a significant concern.[17] Fewer than 8% of practicing US OB-GYNs younger than 50 believed they are able to satisfactorily balance their work and personal lives.[8] When considering a desirable professional practice, OB-GYNs indicated that time for family and personal pursuits, as well as flexible scheduling, were highly important. Those who felt they could control their work and personal lives had higher professional satisfaction scores.[8] One in 4 OB-GYNs younger than 50 was interested in part-time work but did not have this option. Those who wanted to work part-time but could not, were less satisfied professionally.

Nationally, the strongest predictor of work-life balance and burnout is having control over the schedule and hours worked.[7] Overall, OB-GYNs are less satisfied with their careers than other physician specialists. Career satisfaction for OB-GYNs is negatively correlated with working more than 50 hours a week and an uncontrollable schedule, factors that, to date, have practically defined the specialty.[18] Those who do not perform deliveries work fewer hours and have higher career satisfaction.[19] Although physicians who practice obstetrics report enjoying the work, the clinical time they perceive most negatively is being "on-call" on labor and delivery because of the potential of an increased workload and decreased personal control of their schedule.[19]

More Subspecialization

For years, family medicine and obstetrics and gynecology were the 2 major medical specialties with the lowest proportion of residents electing to pursue fellowship training. OB-GYN residents accepted into accredited fellowship programs (reproductive endocrinology and infertility, gynecologic oncology, maternal-fetal medicine) increased from 7.0% in 2000 to 16.5% in 2009.[20] Female pelvic medicine and reconstructive surgery has become an accredited specialty with growing numbers of fellowship programs. In addition, more residents are choosing to enter non–board accredited fellowship training programs in such areas as minimally invasive surgery, family planning and reproductive health, infectious disease, and pediatric and adolescent gynecology.[20]

Although at least 1 in every 4 resident graduates pursues subspecialty training, reasons for this trend in subspecialization have not been studied in depth. We assume that it is a combination of a person's special interest or expertise in a narrower subject, perceived improvement in lifestyle, financial gain, diminished interest in general obstetrics and gynecology, or additive value as a subspecialist in joining a large group practice.[20,21] We anticipate that by 2020, 1 in every 3 residents will undertake some form of subspecialty training.

Larger Practices and Employed Physicians

Surveys of OB-GYN physicians have shown that they are displeased with short times allowed for office visits with inadequate time for counseling and care coordination.[8,22] Many OB-GYNs refer patients to subspecialists, a practice that frustrates them in certain situations, sometimes discourages patients and families, and increases health care costs.

Independent group practices remain the preferred choice for most OB-GYN resident graduates, yet many now prefer to become employed by larger single or multispecialty group practices or hospitals.[21] Some physicians provide only office-based care with or without ambulatory surgery. Female OB-GYNs have consistently elected to retire from practicing obstetrics at mid-career (early or mid-40s) than male OB-GYNs, according to the ACOG Professional Liability surveys.[23]

To accommodate physician lifestyle and conserve overhead costs, small practices are consolidating into larger groups to provide a more predictable workload and on-call hours. We anticipate that larger practices will network into local and regional health care groups in a manner similar to corporations that pioneered technology and efficiency.

Universal Electronic Health Records and Standardizing Health Care

Gains in economies of scale can be learned not only from other health care organizations but also from businesses that excel in data management with electronic technologies and standardization of operations. Use of electronic health records is becoming universal despite limitations that include set-up and maintenance costs, additional physician time, impersonalization of physician-patient interactions, and software packages that are not easy to understand or operate. Electronic records have the potential to provide immediate access to information, support measurement and reporting of outcomes, and enhance more universal standards of care. Physician reporting of resource use, outcome measurements, and cost of care will become an inescapable part of practice management in the future.[24]

The US Department of Health and Human Services, private insurance companies, health systems, and provider networks will be able to specify and track adherence to guidelines for managing patients with various health conditions. When available, evidence-based guidelines have been touted over the past decade as the most appropriate means for clinical care. Patient safety will invariably be improved with more complete information sharing. Portals that document appropriate medical history-taking, telephone calls, adherence to evidence-based treatment protocols, electronic reporting of laboratory results, embedded alerts, and legible records will build a stronger defense against seemingly frivolous and questionable lawsuits.

Emphasis on Quality and Performance Improvement

The Institute of Medicine has called for health systems "to do their work openly; to make their results known to the public and professionals alike; and to build trust through disclosure, even of the systems' own problems."[25] Organizations such as the National Quality Forum, The Joint Commission, Leapfrog Group, large health plans, and The National Priorities Partnership have embraced the Institute's challenge for greater transparency of health care system performance.[24]

OB-GYN practices will be judged on their quality and health care outcomes. Studies have demonstrated that adult patients receive little more than half of recommended evidence-based care.[26] Delivery of care varies between communities, states, and regions, and too often this results in adverse outcomes.[27] Policy makers, employers, purchasers of health care, and consumers are demanding greater accountability. Quality measures are used widely as tools for accountability and for information sharing about caregiver and health system performances. These measures can be used for public reporting, payment incentives, physician maintenance of certification, and value-based purchasing.

Quality improvement can be daunting, yet if we cannot measure outcomes, we cannot begin to manage them. Several areas of obstetrics and gynecology have demonstrated leadership in quality measurement. The American Board of Obstetrics and Gynecology, in collaboration with the ACOG, has a growing focus on measurement and quality improvement. This focus includes quality improvement assignments and required reviews of articles about patient quality and safety as part of an OB-GYN's maintenance of certification. Physicians can advance the field of performance measurement by researching what measures can be collected in their practice, then adding other variables if necessary. Such measures can be based on experiences of either a single patient or cumulative care from either a single physician or team. Hospitals are more likely to partner with providers to assume a greater role in implementing checklists and clinical pathways, particularly if we do not implement those ourselves.

Transformational Forces Leading to Change

Guiding principles that will determine the state of our specialty in the near future result from unprecedented economic, demographic, and workforce pressures that are driving change in health care. Berwick and colleagues[28] at the Institute for Healthcare Improvement developed a simple method of combining these competing needs into a framework known as the "triple aim" of (1) improving the health of the population, (2) obtaining the best experience for the patient, and (3) controlling costs. Any new strategy will not survive unless it can demonstrate overwhelming improvements in clinical outcomes, reductions in costs, or improvements in population health.

External and internal forces have caused an "inflection point" to be reached that requires significant change to the methods of care delivery. In a 3-part series, Lagrew and Jenkins[29–31] divided those significant changes into 4 major "transformational forces." These additive and complementary forces involve (1) payment reform: transitioning away from fee-for-service medicine to value-based care, (2) system reform into team-based medical care, (3) digital conversion of clinical data and health information technology, and (4) disruptive clinical innovations (eg, genomics and epigenetics, minimally invasive therapies, computer-aided diagnoses, and stem-cell therapy and regenerative therapy). Two groups of OB-GYNs are apparent when considering implementing initial changes: transformers who wish to reform medicine into a new world, and preservatives who are incumbents wanting to protect the status quo. Transformers know what to do in sincerely addressing the "triple aim" but are stymied by preservatives.

ROLES OF OBSTETRICIAN-GYNECOLOGIST HOSPITALISTS
Work-Life Balance and Physician Support

Work as an OB-GYN hospitalist holds appeal for women and physicians seeking a better work-life balance, as it meets their needs for reduced or part-time work hours and a more controllable lifestyle. Although any OB-GYN hospitalist program must cover their hospital 24 hours a day, 7 days a week, the number of physicians used to provide this coverage, the number of hours each individual works, and the days and times each physician covers are highly variable. The schedule is often flexible in that each hospitalist often has several days a week when he or she is not providing patient care.

Hours worked and schedules also can be adaptable over an OB-GYN hospitalist's career based on that person's needs and life stage. For example, hospitalists in the childbearing and childrearing years could choose to work fewer hours, but increase the number of hours again at a later life stage if desired. Although the hospitalist position is a partial answer to the demands of an increasingly female OB-GYN workforce for part-time and controllable work, it addresses the needs of any physician who wishes or needs to reduce work hours or control their schedule. Those physicians may be near retirement, restricted by disabilities, or wish to serve in hospital administrative roles.

Another role of the OB-GYN hospitalist would be to become a work-hours extender for generalist or subspecialty colleagues. A group practice could contract with the OB-GYN hospitalists to cover the group's patient rounding responsibilities as well as any admissions on prearranged days, so that members of the group practice would be afforded fewer work hours or on-call shifts. Even subspecialists in maternal-fetal medicine, urogynecology, and gynecologic oncology could reduce their in-house, on-call responsibilities by using OB-GYN hospitalists while providing out-of-hospital and telephone support.

A published survey of OB-GYN hospitalists in 2010 supports variability in scheduling and hours worked, which results in increased satisfaction.[32] Of the OB-GYN hospitalists, 82% were working full-time. Shift length varied between 24 hours (30.8%), 18 hours (8.7%), 12 hours (22.5%), and 8 hours (9.4%). There was much variation in the number of shifts worked per week. Two-thirds of respondents worked 3.5 shifts per week or less, with the common response being 2 shifts (88%). Career satisfaction for OB-GYN hospitalists was quite high. On a scale of −5 (least satisfied) to +5 (most satisfied), 76% of hospitalists answered +3, +4, or +5, whereas only 8% were dissatisfied. This is consistent with previous findings that physicians who worked their preferred number of hours (whether it be full-time or part-time) reported improved job satisfaction, better schedule fit, less burnout, better marital quality, and higher life satisfaction.[3]

Standardization of Care and Quality Improvement

The drive for standardization of care and quality improvement is currently most pronounced in the inpatient setting, where government payment is linked to processes and outcomes. Private payers are not far behind, and hospitals and health care systems are preparing to enter a new era of health care in which goals will be FOCUSED on reducing per capita costs. In these often challenging situations, hospitals turn to their employed physicians to drive practice standardization and improve outcomes for patients and the hospital. Hospitalists, with their focus on inpatient medical care, have become the default champions for hospital standardization and quality improvement.

Given the documented successes of the pediatric and internal medicine hospitalists in improving quality and safety while reducing costs, we must ask if there is a role of the OB-GYN hospitalists in doing the same for our specialty. For example, rates of cesarean deliveries vary broadly by provider, hospital, and state. Standardization of care has the possibility to reduce this rate and accompanying costs. Two recent publications comparing traditional OB-GYN care with OB-GYN hospitalist at 2 different hospitals found that hospitalists reduced the rate of cesarean deliveries.[33,34]

To date, data on OB-GYN hospitalist care are limited with regard to quality, safety, and cost outcomes. However, publications on reduced cesarean rates are encouraging. We predict that OB-GYN hospitalists will continue to drive decreased variations and increase standardization of care in other areas of inpatient obstetrics, such as induction of labor, postpartum hemorrhage, preeclampsia/hypertension, and Category 2 fetal heart rate tracings.

This new era of medicine with increased focuses on inpatient quality, safety, and practice standardization will be accompanied by ever-increasing depth and breadth of information that physicians must integrate and incorporate into their daily practices. OB-GYN hospitalist medicine presents a subspecialization opportunity for those who want to focus professionally on inpatient care, especially in obstetrics, and who are interested in becoming leaders in quality improvement and patient safety.

Between 20% and 50% of maternal deaths in the United States have been deemed preventable through improved quality of care on labor and delivery, including the appropriate diagnosis and recognition of high-risk patients, appropriate and timely treatment, and improved communication to avoid documentation and hand-off errors.[35,36] Six of the 7 most frequent causes of maternal death directly relate to labor, delivery, and immediately postpartum: obstetric hemorrhage, hypertensive disorders, infection, venous thromboembolism, amniotic fluid embolism, and anesthetic complications. Many of these events are sudden and unpredictable, and demand that the attending provider (regardless of specialty) be able to recognize, respond, and treat or call for immediate assistance. Nationwide, OB-GYN hospitalists are becoming the champions for quality and safety in obstetric units, including writing and reinforcing protocols and using checklists to reduce variability of care. An OB-GYN hospitalist is an inpatient obstetric specialist who is an expert in teamwork, communication, simulation, and standardized management of obstetric emergencies.

Although more difficult to assess, severe maternal morbidity may be as high as 100 times more frequent than maternal mortality and "near-miss" obstetric events may complicate up to 0.7% of all deliveries.[37,38] High-frequency, high-hazard adverse events are defined as "areas of relatively frequent error for which effective barriers to prevent the error from reaching the patient are currently suboptimal."[38] The most common errors result from failure of a provider to respond to an immediate patient care need and failure of a provider to follow set safety precautions. The presence of a 24-hour in-house obstetrician with in-depth knowledge and skill to respond to obstetric emergencies, to provide consultative services to midwifery and family medicine colleagues as well as off-campus obstetricians, and to master safety protocols and performance standards according to evidence-based practices should reduce morbidity and mortality.

Financial Considerations

Although patient safety and quality of care remain foremost, OB-GYN hospitalists understand that their program needs to be financially viable. A financially successful program would result from overseeing risk management, reducing operational expense, increasing service revenue, and developing business. Such a program can provide the hospital with more timely coverage to respond to emergent situations and decrease the likelihood of adverse events. This reduction in potential liability can limit overall hospital malpractice exposure. By doing so, some hospitals could reduce their insurance reserves or premium expenses.

Operational expenses may be reduced with an OB-GYN hospitalist program. High-risk situations could be managed without need for a maternal transport, thus minimizing ambulatory care liability. Although hospitalists manage the patient triage process, hospital nurses would be able to concentrate their attention on inpatients.

Service revenue could increase by implementing an OB-GYN hospitalist group program with 24/7 coverage. With such a program, higher-risk pregnancies could be managed without need for maternal transport and perhaps increase in the number of maternal transports into the hospital, which adds business to the intensive care nursery. Hospitalists are inclined to provide more immediate care and prompter decision-making, which can result in more referrals to departments inside and outside the hospital.

Business development may be the strongest advantage of an OB-GYN hospitalist program. The 24/7 coverage can be a positive change for local providers. An OB-GYN hospitalist program has the potential to increase physician retention and recruitment, local clinic partnerships, midwifery group support, any in-house clinics, and maternal transports, which can increase patient volume.

REFERENCES

1. American Medical Association. AMA Physician Masterfile, 2015. Available at: http://www.ama-assn.org/ama/pub/about-ama/physican-data-resources/physician-masterfile.page. Accessed January 22, 2015.
2. Rayburn WF. The obstetrician-gynecologist workforce in the United States: facts, figures, and implications. Washington, DC: American College of Obstetrics and Gynecology; 2011.
3. Pearse WH, Haffner WH, Primack A. Effect of gender on the obstetric-gynecologic work force. Obstet Gynecol 2001;97(5 Pt1):794–7.
4. Promecene PA, Schneider KM, Monga M. Work hours for practicing obstetrician-gynecologists: the reality of life after residency. Am J Obstet Gynecol 2003;189:631–3.
5. Benedetti TJ, Baldwin LM, Andrilla CH, et al. The productivity of Washington state's obstetrician-gynecologist workforce: does gender make a difference? Obstet Gynecol 2004;103:499–505.
6. Reyes JW. Gender gaps in income and productivity of obstetricians and gynecologist. Obstet Gynecol 2007;109:1031–9.
7. Keeton K, Fenner DE, Johnson TR, et al. Predictors of physician career satisfaction, work-life balance, and burnout. Obstet Gynecol 2007;109(4):949–55.

8. Anderson BL, Hale RW, Salsberg E, et al. Outlook for the future of obstetrician-gynecologist workforce. Am J Obstet Gynecol 2008;199:88.e1–8.

9. Jolly S, Griffith KA, DeCastro R, et al. Gender differences in time spent on parenting and domestic responsibilities by high-achieving young physician-researchers. Ann Intern Med 2014;160(5):344–53.

10. Emmons SL, Nichols M, Schulkin J, et al. The influence of physician gender on practice satisfaction among obstetrician gynecologists. Am J Obstet Gynecol 2006;194:1728–38.

11. Dyrbye LN, Shanafelt TD, Balch CM, et al. Relationship between work-home conflicts and burnout among American surgeons: a comparison by sex. Arch Surg 2011;146(2):211–7.

12. Dyrbye LN, Freischlag J, Kaups KL, et al. Work-home conflicts have substantial impact on career decisions that affect the adequacy of the surgical workforce. Arch Surg 2012;147(10):933–9.

13. Schwartz RW, Haley JV, Williams C, et al. The controllable lifestyle factor and students' attitudes about specialty selection. Acad Med 1990;65:207–10.

14. Dorsey ER, Jarjoura D, Rutecki GW. Influence of controllable lifestyle on recent trends in specialty choice by US medical students. JAMA 2003;290(9):1173–8.

15. Dorsey ER, Jarjoura D, Rutecki GW. The influence of controllable lifestyle and sex on the specialty choices of graduating U.S. medical students, 1996-2003. Acad Med 2005;80:791–6.

16. Lambert EM, Holmboe ES. The relationship between specialty choice and gender of U.S. medical students, 1990-2003. Acad Med 2005;80:797–802.

17. Tracy EE, Wiler JL, Holschen JC, et al. Topics to ponder: part-time practice and pay parity. Gend Med 2010;7(4):350–6.

18. Leigh JP, Tancredi DJ, Kravitz RL. Physician career satisfaction within specialties. BMC Health Serv Res 2009;9:166.

19. Bettes BA, Chalas E, Coleman VH, et al. Heavier workload, less personal control: impact of delivery on obstetrician/gynecologists' career satisfaction. Am J Obstet Gynecol 2004;190(3):851–7.

20. Rayburn WF, Grand NF, Gilstrap LC, et al. Pursuit of accredited subspecialties by graduating residents in obstetrics and gynecology, 2000-2012. Obstet Gynecol 2012;120:619–25.

21. Rayburn WF, Strunk AL. Profiles about practicing settings of American College of Obstetricians and Gynecologists Fellows. Obstet Gynecol 2013;122:1295–9.

22. Weinstein L, Wolfe HM. The downward spiral of physician satisfaction: an attempt to avert a crisis within the medical profession. Obstet Gynecol 2007;109:1181–3.

23. Klagholz J, Strunk A. Overview of the 2012 American Congress of Obstetricians and Gynecologists' Survey on Professional Liability. Washington, DC: American College of Obstetricians and Gynecologists; 2012.

24. Glee RE, Winkler R. Quality measurement: what it means for obstetricians and gynecologists. Obstet Gynecol 2013;121:507–10.

25. Institute of Medicine. Crossing the quality chasm: a new health system for the 21st century. Washington, DC: National Academies Press; 2001.

26. McGlynn EA, Asch SM, Adams J, et al. The quality of health care delivered to adults in the United States. N Engl J Med 2003;348:2635–45.

27. Fisher ES, Wennberg JE. Health care quality, geographic variations, and the challenge of supply-sensitive care. Perspect Biol Med 2003;46:69–79.

28. Berwick DM, Nolan TW, Whittington J. The triple aim: care, health, and cost. Health Aff (Millwood) 2008;27:759–69.

29. Lagrew DC Jr, Jenkins TR. The future of obstetrics/gynecology in 2020: a clearer vision. Why is change needed? Am J Obstet Gynecol 2014;211(5):470–4.e1.

30. Lagrew DC Jr, Jenkins TR. The future of obstetrics/gynecology in 2020: a clearer vision: finding true north and the forces of change. Am J Obstet Gynecol 2014; 211(6):617–22.e1.

31. Lagrew DC Jr, Jenkins TR. The future of obstetrics/gynecology in 2020: a clearer vision. Transformational forces and thriving in the new system. Am J Obstet Gynecol 2015;212(1):28–33.e1.

32. Funk C, Anderson BL, Schulkin J, et al. Survey of obstetric and gynecologic hospitalists and laborists. Am J Obstet Gynecol 2010;203:177.e1–4.

33. Iriye BK, Huang WH, Condon J, et al. Implementation of a laborist program and evaluation of the effect upon cesarean delivery. Am J Obstet Gynecol 2013; 209(3):251.e1–6.

34. Nijagal MA, Kuppermann M, Nakagawa S, et al. Two practice models in one labor and delivery unit: association with cesarean delivery rates. Am J Obstet Gynecol 2015;212(4):491.e1–8.

35. Geller SE, Cox SM, Kilpatrick SJ. A descriptive model of preventability in maternal morbidity and mortality. J Perinatol 2006;26(2):79–84.

36. Mitchell C, Lawton E, Morton C, et al. California Pregnancy-Associated Mortality Review: mixed methods approach for improved case identification, cause of death analyses and translation of findings. Matern Child Health J 2014;18(3): 518–26.

37. Callaghan WM, Creanga AA, Kuklina EV. Severe maternal morbidity among delivery and postpartum hospitalizations in the United States. Obstet Gynecol 2012; 120(5):1029–36.

38. Clark SL, Meyers JA, Frye DR, et al. A systematic approach to the identification and classification of near-miss events on labor and delivery in a large, national health care system. Am J Obstet Gynecol 2012;207(6):441–5.

What is an Obstetrics/ Gynecology Hospitalist?

Brigid McCue, MD, PhD*

KEYWORDS

- OB/GYN hospitalist • Patient safety • Obstetric safety program • Work/life balance
- OB/GYN fellowship • Laborist

KEY POINTS

- Obstetrics/gynecology (OB/GYN) hospitalists are at the forefront of efforts to improve patient safety, mitigate challenging work force issues facing OB/GYN, and maintain threatened skill sets.
- Evidence is emerging that programs that include OB/GYN hospitalists decrease the rate of cesarean delivery and preterm birth, increase the rates of trial of labor after cesarean delivery and vaginal birth after cesarean, and maintain scores for patient satisfaction.
- The OB/GYN hospitalist is uniquely positioned to champion the cultural changes in a hospital that lead to the decreased adverse outcomes, malpractice claims, and malpractice payouts.

INTRODUCTION

The obstetrics/gynecology (OB/GYN) hospitalist is the latest subspecialist to evolve from obstetrics and gynecology. Starting in 2002, academic leaders recognized the impact of such coalescing forces as the pressure to reduce maternal morbidity and mortality, stagnant reimbursements and the increasing cost of private practice, decrease in applications for OB/GYN residencies, and the demand among practicing OB/GYNs for work/life balance. Dr Fred Frigoletto and Dr Michael Greene[1] and Dr Louis Weinstein[2] called for adaption of the concept of the internal medicine hospitalist to obstetrics. Initially coined *laborist*, the concept of the OB/GYN hospitalist emerged. Thinking of becoming an OB/GYN hospitalist? Here is what you need to know.

The author reports the following conflict of interest: President of the Society of OB/GYN Hospitalists, a nonprofit professional organization.
Department of Obstetrics and Gynecology, Beth Israel Deaconess Hospital-Plymouth, Plymouth, MA 02339, USA
* 23 Shoe Cottage Lane, Hanover, MA 02339.
E-mail address: bmccue@bidplymouth.org

Obstet Gynecol Clin N Am 42 (2015) 457–461
http://dx.doi.org/10.1016/j.ogc.2015.05.011
0889-8545/15/$ – see front matter © 2015 Elsevier Inc. All rights reserved.

obgyn.theclinics.com

What Is an Obstetrics/Gynecology Hospitalist?

So far this question has no simple answer, which presents an ongoing challenge for hospitalist practice and limits the research opportunities that might clarify the benefits or drawbacks of an OB/GYN hospitalist program. The Society of OB/GYN Hospitalists (SOGH) defines an OB/GYN hospitalist as "an Obstetrician/Gynecologist who has focused their professional practice on care of the hospitalized woman."[3] The OB/GYN hospitalist covers labor and delivery but may also manage consults from the antepartum and postpartum units, the emergency department (ED), and inpatient floors. The term *laborist* is frequently used in reference to OB/GYN hospitalists, and the SOGH defines this practitioner as "an Obstetrician/Gynecologist who has focused their professional practice on the care of pregnant women." Laborist programs minimize distractions that might delay emergency response and rely on alternative call pools for the ED and floor coverage.

The scope of care the OB/GYN hospitalist provides varies considerably from site to site and can include seeing and evaluating all triage patients in an obstetric ED, covering unassigned obstetric patients, back up of community OB/GYN physicians, and support of nonsurgical obstetric providers, such as family medicine physicians and certified nurse midwives. Some OB/GYN hospitalists are maternal fetal medicine (MFM) extenders, managing complex high-risk patients in close collaboration with the MFM physician who is seeing office patients or consulting from home. OB/GYN hospitalists in academic programs supervise resident and medical student education. For the purposes of this discussion, the author uses the encompassing term *OB/GYN hospitalist*, recognizing that the actual scope of practice may vary by site.

In an effort to determine how practicing MFM and OB/GYN physicians define OB/GYN hospitalists, Levine and colleagues surveyed members of the Society for Maternal-Fetal Medicine and the American College of Obstetricians and Gynecologists, asking their definition of the OB/GYN hospitalist. The most consistent answers given were "a physician who is part of a group who provides 24/7 coverage on labor and delivery" (44% of responses) and "an Ob/Gyn who covers unassigned patients (on Labor and Delivery and/or in the ED) and assists other providers for all of their shifts, having no office practice" (24% of responses) (Levine, personal communication, 2015). The concept of the OB/GYN hospitalist subspecialist, without an ambulatory or elective gynecologic surgery practice who focuses on care delivered on labor and delivery, is reflected in the second definition. This role is analogous to that of the internal medicine hospitalist and implies expanded knowledge of hospital systems. Use of standardized protocols and procedures, and adherence to quality measures shown to impact patient safety.[4]

Do Obstetrics/Gynecology Hospitalists Improve Care?

Evidence is emerging that programs that include OB/GYN hospitalists decrease the rate of cesarean delivery and preterm birth, increase the rates of trial of labor after cesarean delivery and vaginal birth after cesarean, and maintain scores for patient satisfaction.[5–7] Comprehensive obstetric safety initiatives, which have included implementation of OB/GYN hospitalist programs at Yale University and New York Presbyterian–Weill Cornell Medical Center achieved substantial reductions in adverse outcomes, malpractice claims, and payouts on malpractice cases.[8,9] Additional components of these initiatives included the use of standardized protocols, obstetric safety nurses, anonymous event reporting, team training and electronic fetal heart rate monitoring certification, and cultural change led by the OB/GYN hospitalist.

How Do Obstetrics/Gynecology Hospitalists Improve Care for an Individual Patient?

Here the OB/GYN hospitalist model diverges from the internal medicine model. Internal medicine hospitalists replace the community internist. Freed from the obligation to admit and round on hospitalized patients, community internists see more office patients, minimize interruptions from floor calls, and reduce scheduling uncertainties. In contrast, OB/GYN hospitalists collaborate with community OB/GYN and MFM physicians. The OB/GYN hospitalist may admit a patient in early labor for the primary obstetrician colleague, augment her labor with Pitocin if needed, interpret a concerning fetal heart tracing, and place internal monitors, all while the patient's primary OB/GYN finishes his or her office or surgical day. The primary OB/GYN then has dinner with his or her family and returns to take charge of the patient for her delivery. The primary OB/GYN might ask the OB/GYN hospitalist to assist at a cesarean section and then for help managing a subsequent postpartum hemorrhage. The OB/GYN hospitalist, having managed several postpartum hemorrhages recently, might place the uterine tamponade balloon and assist with a massive transfusion protocol and then resume care of the patient once she is stabilized, allowing the community OB/GYN to return home. Patients benefit from both the continuity of care with their primary OB/GYN and from the experienced presence of the OB/GYN hospitalist.

How Do Obstetrics/Gynecology Hospitalists Improve Care on a Departmental Level?

The OB/GYN hospitalist is uniquely positioned to champion the cultural changes in a hospital that lead to the decreased adverse outcomes, malpractice claims, and malpractice payouts. Yale defined their OB/GYN hospitalist's role as "... ha(ving) responsibility for the quality of care of the entire obstetric service by providing services to patients within the university practices and emergency backup and consultation for all community physicians."[8] The OB/GYN hospitalist endures compliance with quality measures, such as limiting elective delivery prior to 39 weeks.[10] The use of team training and critical communication tools, such as briefs, huddles, debriefs, and conflict management tools, championed by the OB/GYN hospitalist, increases by the support staff and community OB/GYN physicians and creates a culture of safety. As a surgical assistant, the OB/GYN hospitalist can inform the community OB/GYN physician of evidence-based findings regarding surgical technique and management and encourage continuous learning and quality improvement. OB/GYN hospitalists work defined shifts limiting the detrimental effect of sleep deprivation and increasing enthusiasm for teaching medical students and residents.[11]

What Skills and Educational Background Are Needed to Be a Good Obstetrics/Gynecology Hospitalist?

The collaborative leadership role of the OB/GYN hospitalist requires knowledge, strength of character, excellent communication skills, and an ability to connect and empathize with patients. Do you have what it takes to become an OB/GYN hospitalist?

OB/GYN hospitalists love the practice of obstetrics. They put patients at ease quickly. They commit to extraordinary communication with patients and their families, nurses and support staff, the community OB/GYN, MFM, family medicine, and nurse midwife colleagues, subspecialists, and other hospital staff in the ED, operating room, critical care unit, and blood bank. They show courage in maintaining skills, such as forceps, breech delivery of the second twin, and cesarean hysterectomy. They teach by bringing simulations to their perinatal unit, improving the ability of all of the providers to respond to shoulder dystocia and other obstetric emergencies.[12] They evolve with the literature and commit to evidence-based practice, mentoring other physicians to do the same. They maintain relevant certifications such as board certification, Advanced Cardiac Life Support, Neonatal Resuscitation, and electronic fetal monitoring. They are current regarding the myriad of quality measures and advocate for adherence and accurate reporting. Close collaboration with MFM colleagues facilitates transfers from outside hospitals and increased census in the neonatal ICU.

Can Any Obstetrics/Gynecology Physician Be an Obstetrics/Gynecology Hospitalist?

In the absence of any formal accreditation process, any OB/GYN physician can be an OB/GYN hospitalist. Should any OB/GYN physician be an OB/GYN hospitalist? The potential benefits of comprehensive safety programs rely on OB/GYN hospitalists who are not just shift workers but are mentors and leaders on their perinatal units. The new residency graduate who is awaiting acceptance to fellowship and is looking for a temporary position lacks confidence and experience. The OB/GYN looking to wind down after a long career may lack motivation to assist at a routine cesarean section, teach residents at 3:00 AM, or overcome the resistance from busy nurses to run a mock shoulder dystocia. OB/GYN hospitalists sacrifice their hard-won elective surgical skills and the joy of continuity of primary patient care. There is little predictability on labor and delivery, and the OB/GYN who struggles to make decisions in emergency situations might not consider an OB/GYN hospitalist position. Babies will forever be born at night, and the OB/GYN with an aversion to night calls is poorly suited to the career of the OB/GYN hospitalist.

Are you considering an OB/GYN hospitalist career but need more experience and training? OB/GYN hospitalist fellowships at Winthrop University Hospital and University of California-Irvine are academic opportunities for OB/GYN physicians to build their skill sets, critical care experience, and leadership skills to join or create OB/GYN hospitalist programs. OB/GYN hospitalist staffing agencies are another option for the OB/GYN eager to make a career change but who desires the additional support of a structured program. Reentry is a consideration; the American College of Obstetrics and Gynecology and the American Board of Obstetrics and Gynecology are addressing the challenge of reentry back to office practice or elective gynecologic surgery but lack a defined pathway.

Why Should You Consider Becoming an Obstetrics/Gynecology Hospitalist?

To lead constructive change resulting in improved care for women and their babies is rewarding. To collaborate with your community colleagues in a way that advances their practice and the practice of the entire department, gives much needed call relief, and even prolongs their obstetric career is meaningful. To bring medical students and residents along on your educational journey is affirming. To create a culture whereby all team members, particularly the patients, are valued is empowering. To care for a patient with catastrophic uterine rupture and demonstrate expert communication skills with your team, knowledge of the systems of your unit, and confidence in your clinical skills with a decision-to-incision time of 7 minutes is life affirming, life fulfilling, and lifesaving.

REFERENCES

1. Frigoletto FD, Greene MF. Is there a sea change ahead for obstetrics and gynecology? Obstet Gynecol 2002;100(6):1342–3.
2. Weinstein L. The laborist: a new focus of practice for the obstetrician. Am J Obstet Gynecol 2003;188(2):310–2.
3. SOGH. Availbale at: www.societyofobgynhospitalists.org. 2015.

4. Lindenauer PK, Rothberg MB, Pekow PS, et al. Outcomes of care by hospitalists, general internists, and family physicians. N Engl J Med 2007;357:2589–600.
5. Iriye BK, Huang WH, Condon J, et al. Implementation of a laborist program and evaluation of the effect upon cesarean delivery. Am J Obstet Gynecol 2013; 209(3):251.e1–6.
6. Nijagal MA, Kuppermann M, Nakagawa S, et al. Two practice models in one labor and delivery unit: association with cesarean delivery rates. Am J Obstet Gynecol 2015;212(4):491.e1–8.
7. Srinivas S, Macheras M, Small D, et al. Does the laborist model improve obstetric outcomes? Am J Obstet Gynecol 2013;208(Suppl 1):S48.
8. Pettker CM, Thung SF, Lipkind HS, et al. A comprehensive obstetric patient safety program reduces liability claims and payments. Am J Obstet Gynecol 2014; 211(4):319–25.
9. Grunebaum A, Chervenak F, Skupski D. Effect of a comprehensive obstetric patient safety program on compensation payments and sentinel events. Am J Obstet Gynecol 2011;204(2):97–105.
10. Clark SL, Frye DR, Meyers JA, et al. Reduction in elective delivery at <39 weeks of gestation: comparative effectiveness of 3 approaches to change and the impact on neonatal intensive care admission and stillbirth. Am J Obstet Gynecol 2010;203(5):449.e1–6.
11. Clark SL. Sleep deprivation: implications for obstetric practice in the United States. Am J Obstet Gynecol 2009;201(2):136.e1–4.
12. Draycott TJ, Crofts JF, Ash JP, et al. Improving neonatal outcome through practical shoulder dystocia training. Obstet Gynecol 2008;112(1):14–20.

The Role of Obstetrics/ Gynecology Hospitalists in Reducing Maternal Mortality

Tobey A. Stevens, MD[a],*, Laurie S. Swaim, MD[b],
Steven L. Clark, MD[c]

KEYWORDS

- Maternal morbidity • Maternal mortality • OB/GYN hospitalist
- Postpartum hemorrhage • Hypertensive crisis • Pregnancy-associated hypertension
- Pulmonary edema

KEY POINTS

- Identification of the most preventable causes of maternal mortality and development of processes designed to eliminate common errors found in such cases will lead to fewer maternal deaths.
- Maternal mortality review reveals that significant delay in diagnosis and treatment is a common finding, contributing directly to maternal deaths.
- Obstetrics hospitalists are immediately available to evaluate and treat patients, which could lead to improved patient safety and fewer maternal deaths.
- Postpartum hemorrhage and complications of preeclampsia are significant contributors to maternal morbidity and mortality in the United States. Many of these deaths could be prevented with better communication, faster recognition, coordinated care, and decisive management.

INTRODUCTION

In 2013, 289,000 mothers worldwide lost their lives following pregnancy and childbirth, which equates to 800 women every day. Although 99% of those deaths occurred in developing countries, developed countries, including the United States, are not immune. According to the World Health Organization, 1200 maternal deaths occurred

Conflicts of Interest: The authors report no commercial or financial conflicts of interest related to this article.
[a] Department of Obstetrics & Gynecology, Baylor College of Medicine, 6651 Main Street, Suite1020, Houston, TX 77030, USA; [b] Division of Gynecologic and Obstetric Specialists, Department of Obstetrics and Gynecology, Baylor College of Medicine, 6651 Main Street, Suite 1020, Houston, TX 77030, USA; [c] Maternal Fetal Medicine, Department of Obstetrics and Gynecology, Baylor College of Medicine, 6651 Main Street, Suite 1020, Houston, TX 77030, USA
* Corresponding author.
E-mail address: tasteven@texaschildrens.org

Obstet Gynecol Clin N Am 42 (2015) 463–475
http://dx.doi.org/10.1016/j.ogc.2015.05.005
0889-8545/15/$ – see front matter © 2015 Elsevier Inc. All rights reserved.

obgyn.theclinics.com

in the United States in 2013 (28 per 100,000 live births), representing a 6.1% annual increase in the maternal death rate over the past 13 years.[1]

Although some maternal deaths are not easily preventable, a focus on intrapartum and immediate postpartum causes could result in substantial improvement of this rate. The challenge lies in identifying the preventable causes of maternal mortality so that processes may be implemented with the goal of preventing maternal deaths. The determination of the number of preventable maternal deaths is inexact and varies based on the definition of preventable. Clark and colleagues[2] reviewed maternal outcomes after nearly 1.5 million deliveries at 124 US hospitals and concluded that 17 of the 95 maternal deaths (18%) could have been prevented with more appropriate medical care. Another 10 deaths (11%) were judged to be preventable but occurred as a result of actions or inaction of nonmedical persons.[2] In contrast, Berg and colleague's[3] review of 108 pregnancy-related deaths, which considered the effect of health care system changes and public health infrastructure on the maternal mortality rate, determined that up to 40% of maternal deaths could have been prevented. Regardless of the methods used to define preventable maternal death, by shifting the focus to identification of the most common causes of such deaths and the root cause of each individual occurrence, evidence-based care models can be developed and implemented with the ultimate goal of reducing maternal mortality.

As the maternal mortality has risen, so has acceptance of the hospitalist concept among obstetrician gynecologists and their patients in the United States. The rapid and widespread adoption of obstetrics (OB) hospitalist programs across the United States is evidence of this culture shift. Olson and colleagues[4] reported that in 2012 there were 164 known OB hospitalist programs across the United States, with an average of 2 being added each month. The OB Hospitalist Group, one of the leading consulting and staffing firms in the OB hospitalist industry, reports that as of October 2014 they have designed and installed more than 60 OB hospitalist programs since their inception in 2006, with several more in development. These specific programs span 23 states and have generated 641,869 patient interactions in almost 1.5 million person-hours of coverage.[5] There are also a growing number of OB hospitalist programs at academic institutions across the country. Despite this growing trend, there is a paucity of outcomes data relating specifically to the effect of OB hospitalists on patient care. As a result, of the many advantages offered by hospitalist programs, that of improved patient safety remains unproved.

Given an increasing rate of maternal mortality, exploring ways to reduce maternal mortality through identification of preventable causes is a critical endeavor. Maternal mortality review reveals that significant delay in diagnosis and treatment is a common finding and contributes directly to maternal death.[2] This article examines the role of well-trained OB hospitalists, who are immediately available at the bedside, in improving patient safety and decreasing maternal deaths from preventable causes. Postpartum hemorrhage and complications of preeclampsia are among the most common causes of preventable maternal deaths in the United States. This article examines both. In each case, the appropriate course of action, common pitfalls in patient care, and ultimately how the availability of a well-trained, experienced OB hospitalist might negate a catastrophic outcome are explored.

POSTPARTUM HEMORRHAGE
Background

Despite numerous medical advances and an increased awareness, postpartum hemorrhage remains a significant cause of maternal morbidity and mortality in the United

States. In an analysis of 115,502 women who delivered between 2008 and 2011, Grobman and colleagues[6] found that postpartum hemorrhage was responsible for approximately half of all severe maternal morbidity. According to the most recent data from the US Centers for Disease Control and Prevention[7] (CDC), about 11.3% of all US obstetric deaths are caused by hemorrhage and the rate of postpartum hemorrhage seems to be increasing. Bateman and colleagues[8] reviewed the Nationwide Inpatient Sample (NIS), which is the largest publicly available inpatient health care database in the United States, and found that the overall rate of postpartum hemorrhage increased 27.5% between 1995 and 2004, primarily because of an increase in the incidence of uterine atony, which accounted for 79% of those cases. In that same series, postpartum hemorrhage was associated with 19.1% of all in-hospital deaths after delivery. Callaghan and colleague's[9] review of the NIS further echoed these findings. The percentage of deliveries with an International Classification of Diseases, Ninth Revision, Clinical Modification (ICD-9-CM) code for postpartum hemorrhage increased by 26% between 1994 and 2006 and the rate of hemorrhage caused by uterine atony increased by 50%, from 1.6% to 2.4% over that same time span. In a more recent review of the NIS from 1998 to 2009 Callaghan and colleagues[10] noted that the number of women requiring blood transfusion at time of delivery admission is increasing, with an increase from 34.04 per 10,000 delivery hospitalizations in 1998 to 96.38 per 10,000 delivery hospitalizations in 2008. Mhyre and colleagues[11] reviewed the State Inpatient Dataset for New York (1998–2007) and found that massive blood transfusion, the hallmark of significant obstetric hemorrhage, was strongly associated with in-hospital maternal death, with a mortality frequency of 3.4% compared with 1 in 10,000 in the general delivery population.

The data is clear: obstetric hemorrhage is a substantial and growing challenge for obstetric providers in the United States. However, many, if not most, maternal deaths from hemorrhage are preventable. Between 2000 and 2006, Clark and colleagues[2] performed a system-wide review of 1,461,270 deliveries across the Hospital Corporation of America system. During that time, 8 of 11 maternal deaths attributed to hemorrhage were judged to be preventable. Similarly, in Berg and colleagues'[3] review of 108 pregnancy-related deaths, 93% of the deaths caused by hemorrhage were thought to be preventable. Given the increasing frequency of postpartum hemorrhage and the preventable nature of the associated morbidity and mortality, priority should be placed on exploring practices designed to reduce this burden. Early involvement of experienced practitioners is essential in the event of severe and ongoing maternal hemorrhage. By virtue of their continuous care of laboring patients, active involvement in hospital safety initiatives, and immediate availability, obstetric hospitalists are specifically trained to manage such emergencies.

Preparation

Appropriate preparation is the cornerstone of successful postpartum hemorrhage management. When referring to postpartum hemorrhage, the American College of Obstetricians and Gynecologists (ACOG) suggests that, "All obstetric units and practitioners must have the facilities, personnel, and equipment in place to manage this emergency properly."[12] Identification of maternal risk factors for postpartum hemorrhage and tailoring care to the patient's relative risk are critical components of preparation. However, a large proportion of women who develop postpartum hemorrhage do not have any identifiable risk factors. Furthermore, even in the largest delivery centers, the absolute number of patients experiencing severe obstetric hemorrhage and massive blood transfusion is low, and many providers have limited experience with these rare and intense situations. Mhyre and colleagues'[11] findings showed that

0.06% of patients received 10 or more units of blood for obstetric hemorrhage at time of delivery hospitalization. In a center performing 10,000 deliveries a year, their experience would be just 1 massive transfusion every 2 months. This finding underscores the importance of both institutional preparedness and the availability of on-site, well-trained physicians and staff. Clinical simulations and multidisciplinary protocols are the foundations of preparation. The Joint Commission on Accreditation has recommended both and the literature clearly supports this recommendation. Shields and colleagues[13] found that, at the institutional level, adoption of a comprehensive maternal hemorrhage protocol led to resolution of bleeding at an earlier stage, use of fewer blood products, and a reduced rate of disseminated intravascular coagulation (DIC). When similar protocols were implemented across a larger health care system, Shields and colleagues[14] noted a 25.9% reduction per 1000 births in the use of blood products and a 14.8% reduction in the number of patients who underwent peripartum hysterectomy for obstetric hemorrhage. The algorithm for primary postpartum hemorrhage used at our institution is shown in **Fig. 1**. Protocols such as this allow clinicians to focus on steps in an algorithm rather than recall from memory, which often fails them in situations of extreme stress. This approach leads to more coordinated care and improved patient outcomes. Likewise, frequent protocol simulations provide the opportunity to improve team communication and identify commonly encountered clinical and logistical barriers to optimal patient care. This type of experiential learning, when done on a regular basis, converts a rare and potentially life-threatening situation into a coordinated routine that can improve outcome.

The role of obstetric hospitalists is to spearhead these lifesaving initiatives with nursing and administrative leaders. Practicing obstetricians are often at offsite care facilities, or scrubbed in surgery. Some have small obstetric practices or fewer years of experience. When selected appropriately, OB/(GYN) hospitalists also have the benefit of significant past clinical experience, are on site, and are frequently the first responders in emergency situations. According to a recent survey by ObGynHospitalist.com, most hospitalists are between 40 and 59 years of age and are at least 6 years postresidency.[15] A trained obstetric hospitalist with the ability to respond to obstetric emergencies is an invaluable resource to patients, hospitals, and providers. OB hospitalists also coordinate care with all team members, whereas primary providers tend to their own patients.

Recognition and Initial Measures

Effective management of obstetric hemorrhage begins with accurate determination of blood loss and rapid initiation of initial interventions. Although training can help, visual estimation of blood loss is commonly underestimated by as much as 30% to 50%.[16] Communication is often a barrier to recognition as well. The nurse caring for the patient often verbally describes the estimated blood loss to a physician over the phone, which makes it difficult for the physician to accurately gauge the degree of bleeding and the patient's clinical condition. In this situation, the OB/GYN hospitalist could be at the bedside within minutes, offering a direct estimation of blood loss and assessment of the patient's clinical status, and acting as an extension of the primary provider. The hospitalist then clearly communicates the level of urgency with the patient's physician and is on hand to initiate care immediately. This degree of rapid response is paramount in the setting of significant ongoing obstetric hemorrhage. After ensuring adequate intravenous access and supporting the patient's oxygenation, prompt bedside evaluation and bimanual examination by the obstetrician should follow. In Driessen and colleagues'[17] review of postpartum hemorrhage after vaginal deliveries, severe postpartum hemorrhage was 1.8 times higher when bimanual

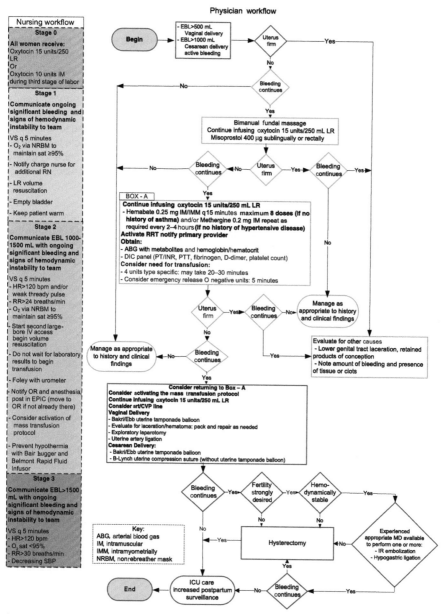

Fig. 1. Texas Children's Hospital evidence-based outcomes center clinical algorithm for primary postpartum hemorrhage (PPH) caused by uterine atony. ABG, Arterial Blood Gas; Art, arterial; bpm, beats per minute; CVP, central venous pressure; EBL, estimated blood loss; EPIC, electronic medical record; HR, heart rate; ICU, intensive care unit; IM, Intramuscular; IMM, Intramyometrially; INR, International Normalized Ratio; IR, interventional radiology; LR, lactated Ringer; MD, Doctor of Medicine; NRBM, Non-Rebreather Mask; OR, operating room; PT, prothrombin time; PTT, partial thromboplastin time; q, every; RN, registered nurse; RR, respiratory rate; RRT, rapid response team; sat, saturation; SBP, systolic blood pressure; VS, vital signs.

examination occurred more than 20 minutes after the diagnosis of postpartum hemorrhage compared with bimanual examination within the first 10 minutes after diagnosis. In the same analysis, risk of severe postpartum hemorrhage was 1.6 times higher when the call for obstetric assistance was delayed compared with cases in which a senior obstetrician was present or called within 10 minutes of the diagnosis.[17]

Delay in accurate diagnosis and delay in initiation of treatment are the two most common preventable errors in cases of ongoing obstetric hemorrhage secondary to uterine atony. Both increase the likelihood of significant maternal morbidity and ultimately mortality. When a morbidly adherent placenta is the source of bleeding, failure to recognize and adequately prepare in advance is the most common pitfall. This article focuses on those cases that do not involve abnormal placentation, although, once ongoing bleeding is present, many of the same principles apply regardless of the cause.

Diagnosis and Definitive Management

Obstetric hemorrhage is a sign not a diagnosis. Clinicians must immediately begin searching for a cause as soon as postpartum hemorrhage is recognized. Supportive care is provided while the diagnostic phase is ongoing. Prompt attention to diagnosis and support are imperative, thus hospitalists are perfectly positioned as the first responders in such situations. When atony is present, manual massage is performed, the bladder is drained, and uterotonics are used. All of this can take place while the primary physician is en route to the bedside. If atony is found not to be the source, a stepwise approach to determining the cause can follow. All of this coincides with close monitoring of the patient's clinical status and, if available, pertinent laboratory data. Once the primary provider arrives there is a collaborative effort between the hospitalist and the patient's provider. The hospitalist is able to coordinate other services and ancillary staff because of a clear understanding of institutional protocols. If initial conservative measures fail to control bleeding secondary to uterine atony the clinician's sense of urgency must be increased. The thought process of all involved should transition from that of a normal delivery situation to that of a life-threatening emergency. Blood and component therapy should be considered if not already initiated, and moving the patient to the operating suite should be considered earlier rather than later. In a review of common mistakes made during simulation-based postpartum hemorrhage training, Maslovitz and colleagues[18] found that 2 of the most common errors were delay in transporting the patient to the operating room and delay in administration of blood products to reverse consumptive coagulopathy. If balloon tamponade was not attempted in the delivery room it should be considered here. There will either be rapid confirmation of hemostasis or the bleeding will continue to occur around or into the device, necessitating other measures. The balloon can also function as a temporizing measure while en route to the operating suite or while preparations for laparotomy are being made. Selective arterial embolization should be considered only if the patient is experiencing low-grade ongoing bleeding and is clinically stable. This technique, which requires specialized equipment and staff, can delay definitive management. For that reason arterial embolization is of no value in the setting of acute, massive postpartum bleeding.[19] A patient who is not stable enough to withstand such delays should undergo immediate laparotomy.

Failure to rapidly move toward definitive surgical treatment in patients with ongoing postpartum hemorrhage after ineffective medical therapy results in preventable maternal morbidity and death. If conservative measures have failed to control bleeding within 15 to 30 minutes, or if the patient becomes unstable, invasive measures must follow.[20] At the time of laparotomy, many techniques are at the clinician's disposal. The primary provider may have limited experience or be unfamiliar with some of these options. The hospitalist assists the primary provider to work efficiently and methodically through clinical decision making toward laparotomy. Once laparotomy commences, obstetric hospitalists are well versed in intraoperative management techniques for postpartum hemorrhage, including uterine compression sutures, uterine artery ligation, and peripartum hysterectomy. Initial measures include inspection of the uterus with repair of any defects that are found. If atony is the source, the tamponade test followed by various types of uterine compression sutures can be deployed. Next, selective arterial ligation can be attempted. Although hypogastric artery ligation is being performed less frequently, bilateral uterine artery ligation (O'Leary sutures) can accomplish the same goal. O'Leary sutures are generally faster and technically easier. The utero-ovarian ligaments can be ligated as well in an attempt to further diminish blood flow to the uterus. When uncontrollable postpartum hemorrhage persists, prudent obstetricians proceed with rapid hysterectomy. This decision can be difficult but it is a decision that must be made without delay when the patient's life is at stake. Ideally, the decision should be made by the most experienced obstetrician present and supported by a second, if possible.[21]

Summary

Significant obstetric hemorrhage can have catastrophic consequences. Delayed recognition, indecisive management, and disorganized care are three common factors that increase the likelihood of severe maternal morbidity and mortality. However, with thorough preparation, rapid recognition, methodical treatment, and a coordinated multidisciplinary approach, many tragic outcomes can be avoided. On-site, experienced OB hospitalists are able to intervene and facilitate at each stage of patient care and can be an integral part of improving patient outcomes in cases of significant obstetric hemorrhage.

COMPLICATIONS OF PREECLAMPSIA
Background

Hypertensive disorders of pregnancy, including preeclampsia, complicate 5% to 10% of all pregnancies. The prevalence of hypertensive disorders among patients admitted for delivery is increasing, and the related complications remain among the major causes of maternal morbidity and mortality in the United States.[22] In Grobman and colleagues'[6] cohort of more than 100,000 women who delivered between 2008 and 2011, hypertensive complications accounted for 20.5% of severe maternal morbidity, second only to postpartum hemorrhage.[6] According to the CDC's Pregnancy Mortality Surveillance data, hypertensive disorders of pregnancy accounted for 9.4% of the pregnancy-related deaths between 2006 and 2010.[7] In Clark and colleagues'[2] review of nearly 1.5 million deliveries at Hospital Corporation of America (HCA) facilities between 2000 and 2006, 15.8% of 95 maternal deaths were attributed to complications of preeclampsia. Berg and colleague's[3] review of 105 pregnancy-related deaths in North Carolina found that 10% were caused by pregnancy-induced hypertension. Another 9% of the deaths were attributed to cerebrovascular accidents.[3]

Because hypertension-related maternal deaths are among those recognized as being most preventable, many of the adverse outcomes related to hypertensive disorders can be avoided with appropriate recognition and management. In Clark and colleagues'[2] review, approximately 30% of the maternal deaths caused by complications of preeclampsia were potentially preventable, whereas Berg and colleague's[3] deemed 60% of deaths attributed to pregnancy-induced hypertension in their series to be preventable.

Three key errors are commonly seen when preventable preeclampsia-related deaths occur. First, there may be an inappropriate response to, or failure to evaluate, abnormal blood pressures in the clinic setting. Second, there may be an improper response to, or failure to respond to, severe hypertension. Third, there may be a failure to recognize and treat pulmonary edema.[23] Whether the patient is presenting antepartum, intrapartum, or postpartum, dedicated OB hospitalists are uniquely and immediately available to evaluate and treat peripartum patients with complications of hypertension in a timely fashion. The presence of the OB hospitalist is pivotal in the management of 2 life-threatening complications of preeclampsia: acute hypertensive crisis and new-onset pulmonary edema.

Acute Hypertensive Crisis

Background
Cerebral hemorrhage is a complication of severely increased blood pressure and can result in irreversible neurologic damage or sudden death. Cerebral hemorrhage remains a leading cause of death in women with preeclampsia despite the availability of effective antihypertensive medications.[2] Mackay and colleagues[24] reviewed the CDC's Pregnancy Mortality Surveillance system data from 1972 to 1992 and found that 38.7% of the preeclampsia-related maternal deaths were caused by cerebrovascular complications, primarily cerebrovascular hemorrhage. In another series of 28 patients who sustained a stroke in association with severe preeclampsia and eclampsia, the mortality was 53.6%, and only 3 of those who survived did not have long-term morbidity.[25]

Recognition and management
Delays in recognition, diagnosis, and treatment are consistent findings among detailed case reviews of hypertension-related maternal deaths. Specifically, such reviews have noted that untreated blood pressure, significantly exceeding 160/110 mm Hg just before the event, is a common finding.[18] ACOG defines a hypertensive emergency as acutely occurring hypertension, persisting for greater than 15 minutes, and presenting in a pregnant or postpartum patient with preeclampsia or eclampsia.[26] Patients with severe-range blood pressures and/or symptoms require prompt recognition, immediate evaluation, and timely treatment in order to prevent permanent end-organ damage, namely stroke and its sequelae.

For these reasons, an aggressive approach to blood pressure control is prudent, and rapid evaluation and management are critical in the setting of hypertensive crisis. Protocols for antihypertensive therapy have been implemented and have been successful.[27,28] The success of such protocols is enhanced by the caveats listed in **Box 1**.

Box 1
Successful protocols

- Should be highly specific to the disorder
- Should be instituted rapidly
- Should be instituted automatically once diagnosis made, without the need for additional physician orders

Data from Clark SL, Christmas JT, Frye DR, et al. Maternal mortality in the United States: predictability and the impact of protocols on fatal postcesarean pulmonary embolism and hypertension-related intracranial hemorrhage. Am J Obstet Gynecol 2014;211(1):32.e31–9; and von Dadelszen P, Sawchuck D, McMaster R, et al. The active implementation of pregnancy hypertension guidelines in British Columbia. Obstet Gynecol 2010;116(3):659–66.

In a retrospective evaluation, Clark and colleagues[27] noted a reduction in preeclampsia-associated maternal death from 15 during the 7-year preimplementation period to 3 during the 6 years after implementation of an HCA-wide (110 facilities) Hypertension Management Protocol, as shown in **Box 2**. After protocol implementation, deaths from in-hospital intracranial hemorrhage were eliminated.[27] von Dadelszen and colleagues[28] performed a preintervention and postintervention cohort comparison after introduction of a pregnancy hypertension guideline in Canada. They examined the British Columbia Perinatal Database Registry and found that, in the 2 years following guideline implementation, the incidence of combined adverse maternal outcomes related to hypertension decreased from 3.1% to 1.9%.[28]

When predetermined blood pressure thresholds have been exceeded, an institutional protocol for the management of hypertensive crisis enables bedside caretakers to begin acute management without awaiting the arrival of the evaluating clinician the bedside. Initial evaluation should be the same regardless of the underlying cause of the acute hypertension. Once the physician arrives, the patient is triaged promptly after a focused and pertinent review of cardiovascular, neurologic, and respiratory

---

Box 2
Blood pressure management of severe intrapartum or postpartum hypertension using hydralazine

Use of this protocol is one way for a clinician to be in full compliance with the existing standard of care as it applied to this issue. Alternative approaches exist that are equally acceptable.

The following protocol should be initiated if the systolic blood pressure is greater than or equal to 160 mm Hg or the diastolic blood pressure is greater than or equal to 110 mm Hg:

- Notify physician
- Administer hydralazine 5 mg intravenously (IV) over 2 minutes
- Repeat blood pressure in 15 minutes
- If either blood pressure threshold is still exceeded, administer hydralazine 10 mg IV over 2 minutes
- Repeat blood pressure in 15 minutes
- If either blood pressure threshold is still exceeded, administer labetalol 20 mg IV over 2 minutes
- Repeat blood pressure in 10 minutes
- If either blood pressure criteria is still exceeded, administer labetalol 40 mg IV over 2 minutes and obtain emergency maternal-fetal medicine, internal medicine, or anesthesia consultation regarding blood pressure control
- Repeat blood pressure in 10 minutes
- Additional medication per specific order
- Once the blood pressure thresholds are achieved, repeat blood pressure every 10 minutes for 1 hour, then every 15 minutes for 1 hour, then every 30 minutes for 1 hour, then blood pressures every hour for 4 hours
- Additional blood pressure timing per specific order

Similar protocols exist for the use of labetalol and nifedipine.

From Clark SL, Christmas JT, Frye DR, et al. Maternal mortality in the United States: predictability and the impact of protocols on fatal postcesarean pulmonary embolism and hypertension-related intracranial hemorrhage. Am J Obstet Gynecol 2014;211(1):32.e31–9, Hospital Corporation of America; with permission.

symptoms. A more thorough medical history then follows along with a physical examination focusing on end-organ damage. However, the patient's private physician may not be available because of other patient care responsibilities. In these critical circumstances, OB hospitalists serve a crucial role. Because of near instant availability, the hospitalist is positioned to evaluate the patient and facilitate potentially lifesaving treatment immediately. This early intervention has the potential to alleviate the crisis before the arrival of the patient's private physician.

Multiple factors contribute to delays in diagnosis and management, which would improve with the availability of obstetric hospitalists. For example, the hospitalist erases the time lag that occurs when nurses await responses from attending providers. Clark states that: "No hospitalized pregnant woman with a blood pressure of either 160 systolic or 110 diastolic will be harmed by a single intravenous bolus of 5–10 mg of hydralazine or 20 mg of labetalol. Yet, many women will benefit."[19] However, because of lack of experience or knowledge, there may be confusion about the timing of repeat blood pressure readings and the administration of therapeutic agents. Reasonable intervals between medication doses and a clear understanding of pharmacokinetics in pregnant hypertensive women are necessary in order to reduce the blood pressure to a safe range while avoiding hypotension that could affect uteroplacental blood flow. The management of hypertensive crisis is another example of a clinical emergency whereby a readily available OB hospitalist and a well-versed care team armed with disease-specific, evidence-based protocols to guide treatment can eliminate confusion and ultimately improve outcomes.

Pulmonary Edema

Background

Acute pulmonary edema is uncommon in normal pregnancies. Sciscione and colleagues[29] reviewed 62,917 consecutive pregnancies delivered at a single institution between 1989 and 1999 and found that pulmonary edema complicated only 51 (0.08%). Compared with healthy pregnant women, those with preeclampsia are at an increased risk of developing pulmonary edema. The mechanisms behind which preeclampsia leads to pulmonary edema include endothelial damage, decreased colloid osmotic pressure, left ventricular dysfunction, and increased peripheral vascular resistance. As a result, acute pulmonary edema can occur in up to 3% of women with preeclampsia, most of which occur in the postpartum period.[30] In Grobman and colleagues'[6] cohort of more than 100,000 parturients, acute cardiopulmonary complications, including pulmonary edema, accounted for 19% of severe maternal morbidity.

Recognition and management

Undiagnosed pulmonary edema is a leading cause of preventable maternal death,[2] and represents a form of acute cardiac failure that should trigger an immediate emergency response. Morbidity is increased when reports of shortness of breath are not taken seriously or evaluated promptly. Pregnant or postpartum women with preeclampsia and complaints of shortness of breath, hypoxemia as shown by decreased O_2 saturation on pulse oximetry, persistent cough, or acute increase in respiratory rate should trigger prompt evaluation. Such a response is not possible if the patient's attending physician is not present in the hospital. The clinical status of patients experiencing acute pulmonary edema can deteriorate rapidly, and delays in diagnosis and initiation of treatment can be fatal. Therefore, the ability of the bedside nurse to rapidly engage an experienced OB hospitalist can be pivotal in the prevention of adverse sequelae in this setting. The hospitalist is able to principally manage the acute pulmonary issues, evaluate, treat, and provide supportive care until arrival, and hand off to the patient's primary physician.

Initial evaluation of patients with acute hypoxemia and/or respiratory distress includes a 12 lead electrocardiogram and close trending of blood pressure, oxygen saturation, respiratory rate, temperature, and fluid balance. In this setting, expeditious imaging with a chest radiograph is also recommended. Most obstetricians have limited experience with auscultation of rales; therefore, a physical finding of clear lungs is often insufficient when the risk of pulmonary edema is high. A chest radiograph is simple, quick, inexpensive, and detects all cases of potentially life-threatening pulmonary edema.[19] In most instances a portable 1-view chest radiograph is adequate. While awaiting the results of imaging studies, simultaneous supportive care with supplemental oxygen can be optimized. If clinical suspicion is high, intravenous furosemide (20 mg–40 mg) should be used to promote diuresis. An experienced care team including maternal-fetal medicine, anesthesia, and critical care staff can be assembled if needed. After the patient is stabilized, an echocardiogram may be indicated to evaluate for significant cardiac dysfunction. A ventilation perfusion scan or spiral computed tomography should be pursued in the setting of arterial hypoxemia in a pregnant or peripartum patient and negative chest radiograph.

Summary

Pregnancies complicated by preeclampsia are common and usually conclude with a healthy mother and child. However, clinicians must remain vigilant for worsening preeclampsia and its consequences. Preeclampsia-related maternal deaths continue to occur in the United States despite a wealth of available diagnostic studies and therapeutic agents. Many of these deaths may be preventable and could potentially be avoided with timely and appropriate medical intervention. Hypertensive crisis and acute pulmonary edema are life-threatening sequelae of preeclampsia. In both instances, expeditious evaluation and management are paramount. When the patient's primary physician is not readily available, an experienced OB hospitalist can intervene immediately, potentially avoiding many tragic outcomes.

SUMMARY

Maternal deaths remain a rare occurrence in the United States but maternal mortality has increased in recent years.[1] Severe maternal morbidity during delivery hospitalization seems to be increasing as well, more than doubling between 1998 and 2011.[10] Although maternal deaths from hemorrhage and hypertensive disorders of pregnancy have trended down in the United States in recent years, they remain common causes of preventable maternal death. In Creanga and colleagues'[31] recent review of the Pregnancy Mortality Surveillance System (2006–2010), hemorrhage, hypertensive disorders, and cerebrovascular accidents accounted for a combined 27% of all pregnancy-related deaths.

Maternal deaths attributed to these causes are among those recognized as being most preventable. Delays in recognition, evaluation, diagnosis, and treatment are consistent findings among detailed case reviews of maternal deaths caused by peripartum hemorrhage and complications of preeclampsia. Evidence-based hemorrhage protocols and guidelines to direct care in the event of acute hypertensive crisis are well supported and seem to be improving outcomes; however, the value of prompt bedside evaluation by an experienced physician cannot be overstated.

In the event of significant peripartum hemorrhage, hypertensive crisis, or acute pulmonary edema, early involvement of an experienced practitioner is essential to optimal patient outcomes. OB hospitalists are immediately available and should have significant past clinical experience. These physicians are uniquely positioned to intervene and facilitate at every stage of patient care. If used properly, OB hospitalists are a valuable resource in the effort to decrease maternal morbidity and mortality.

REFERENCES

1. WHO, UNICEF, UNFPA, The World Bank and the United Nations Population Division. Trends in maternal mortality: 1990-2013. Available at: http://www.who.int/reproductivehealth/publications/monitoring/maternal-mortality-2013/en/. Accessed September 1, 2014.
2. Clark SL, Belfort MA, Dildy GA, et al. Maternal death in the 21st century: causes, prevention, and relationship to cesarean delivery. Am J Obstet Gynecol 2008; 199(1):36.e31–5 [discussion: 91–2.e7–11].
3. Berg CJ, Harper MA, Atkinson SM, et al. Preventability of pregnancy-related deaths: results of a state-wide review. Obstet Gynecol 2005;106(6):1228–34.
4. Olson R, Garite TJ, Fishman A, et al. Obstetrician/gynecologist hospitalists: can we improve safety and outcomes for patients and hospitals and improve lifestyle for physicians? Am J Obstet Gynecol 2012;207(2):81–6.
5. OB Hospitalist Group. Program overview. Available at: http://www.obhg.com/program-overview/metrics. Accessed September 1, 2014.
6. Grobman WA, Bailit JL, Rice MM, et al. Frequency of and factors associated with severe maternal morbidity. Obstet Gynecol 2014;123(4):804–10.
7. Centers for Disease Control and Prevention. Pregnancy-related mortality surveillance. 2014. Available at: http://www.cdc.gov/reproductivehealth/MaternalInfantHealth/PMSS.html. Accessed September 1, 2014.
8. Bateman BT, Berman MF, Riley LE, et al. The epidemiology of postpartum hemorrhage in a large, nationwide sample of deliveries. Anesth Analg 2010;110(5): 1368–73.
9. Callaghan WM, Kuklina EV, Berg CJ. Trends in postpartum hemorrhage: United States, 1994-2006. Am J Obstet Gynecol 2010;202(4):353.e351–6.
10. Callaghan WM, Creanga AA, Kuklina EV. Severe maternal morbidity among delivery and postpartum hospitalizations in the United States. Obstet Gynecol 2012; 120(5):1029–36.
11. Mhyre JM, Shilkrut A, Kuklina EV, et al. Massive blood transfusion during hospitalization for delivery in New York State, 1998-2007. Obstet Gynecol 2013; 122(6):1288–94.
12. American College of Obstetricians and Gynecologists. ACOG practice bulletin: clinical management guidelines for obstetrician-gynecologists number 76, October 2006: postpartum hemorrhage. Obstet Gynecol 2006;108(4):1039–47.
13. Shields LE, Smalarz K, Reffigee L, et al. Comprehensive maternal hemorrhage protocols improve patient safety and reduce utilization of blood products. Am J Obstet Gynecol 2011;205(4):368.e361–8.
14. Shields LE, Wiesner S, Fulton J, et al. Comprehensive maternal hemorrhage protocols reduce the use of blood products and improve patient safety. Am J Obstet Gynecol 2015;212(3):272–80.
15. ObGynHospitalist.com. "Salary and employment survey summary 2014." Available at: http://www.obgynhospitalist.com/topics/61/threads/144. Accessed July 28, 2014.
16. Dildy GA, Paine AR, George NC, et al. Estimating blood loss: can teaching significantly improve visual estimation? Obstet Gynecol 2004;104(3):601–6.

17. Driessen M, Bouvier-Colle MH, Dupont C, et al. Postpartum hemorrhage resulting from uterine atony after vaginal delivery: factors associated with severity. Obstet Gynecol 2011;117(1):21–31.
18. Maslovitz S, Barkai G, Lessing JB, et al. Recurrent obstetric management mistakes identified by simulation. Obstet Gynecol 2007;109(6):1295–300.
19. Clark SL, Hankins GD. Preventing maternal death: 10 clinical diamonds. Obstet Gynecol 2012;119(2.1):360–4.
20. Haeri S, Dildy GA. Maternal mortality from hemorrhage. Semin Perinatol 2012; 36(1):48–55.
21. Abdul-Kadir R, McLintock C, Ducloy AS, et al. Evaluation and management of postpartum hemorrhage consensus from an international expert panel. Transfusion 2014;54(7):1756–68.
22. Kuklina EV, Ayala C, Callaghan WM. Hypertensive disorders and severe obstetric morbidity in the United States. Obstet Gynecol 2009;113(6):1299–306.
23. Clark SL. Strategies for reducing maternal mortality. Semin Perinatol 2012; 36(1):42–7.
24. MacKay AP, Berg CJ, Atrash HK. Pregnancy-related mortality from preeclampsia and eclampsia. Obstet Gynecol 2001;97(4):533–8.
25. Martin JN Jr, Thigpen BD, Moore RC, et al. Stroke and severe preeclampsia and eclampsia: a paradigm shift focusing on systolic blood pressure. Obstet Gynecol 2005;105(2):246–54.
26. American College of Obstetricians and Gynecologists. Committee opinion number 514: emergent therapy for acute-onset, severe hypertension with preeclampsia and eclampsia. Obstet Gynecol 2011;118(6):1465–8.
27. Clark SL, Christmas JT, Frye DR, et al. Maternal mortality in the United States: predictability and the impact of protocols on fatal postcesarean pulmonary embolism and hypertension-related intracranial hemorrhage. Am J Obstet Gynecol 2014;211(1):32.e31–9.
28. von Dadelszen P, Sawchuck D, McMaster R, et al. The active implementation of pregnancy hypertension guidelines in British Columbia. Obstet Gynecol 2010; 116(3):659–66.
29. Sciscione AC, Ivester T, Largoza M, et al. Acute pulmonary edema in pregnancy. Obstet Gynecol 2003;101(3):511–5.
30. Dennis AT, Solnordal CB. Acute pulmonary oedema in pregnant women. Anaesthesia 2012;67(6):646–59.
31. Creanga AA, Berg CJ, Syverson C, et al. Pregnancy-related mortality in the United States, 2006-2010. Obstet Gynecol 2015;125(1):5–12.

Impact of Obstetrician/Gynecologist Hospitalists on Quality of Obstetric Care (Cesarean Delivery Rates, Trial of Labor After Cesarean/Vaginal Birth After Cesarean Rates, and Neonatal Adverse Events)

CrossMark

Brian K. Iriye, MD

KEYWORDS

- Hospitalist • Laborist • Cesarean delivery • VBAC • TOLAC • Value-based care

KEY POINTS

- Obstetric hospitalist programs are increasing rapidly in the United States, providing 24-hour in-hospital coverage in attempts to improve patient safety and quality.
- Full-time obstetric hospitalist programs reduce cesarean delivery rates.
- Obstetric hospitalist coverage improves the rate of trial of labor after cesarean/vaginal birth after cesarean.
- Full-time obstetric hospitalist coverage is a cost-effective solution for coverage of a labor and delivery unit and appears to add value to women's health care.
- Further research is needed on maternal and neonatal outcomes to confirm the initial promising results of the obstetric hospitalist model.

INTRODUCTION

The era of the hospitalist model in obstetric care is currently progressing through its initial stages. From the early formation of the hospitalist movement in the 1990s, to the further thoughts of Weinstein on "laborists" in 2003, and now the initial outcome studies of these programs, the obstetric hospitalist movement has gained acceptance inside the realm of maternal health.[1,2] Within other specialties, the hospitalist concept inched forward and expanded without specific initial plans for measuring quality and

Disclosures: The author has no conflicts of interest to disclose.
High Risk Pregnancy Center, 2011 Pinto Lane, Suite 200, Las Vegas, NV 89106, USA
E-mail address: bki@hrpregnancy.com

Obstet Gynecol Clin N Am 42 (2015) 477–485
http://dx.doi.org/10.1016/j.ogc.2015.05.006
0889-8545/15/$ – see front matter © 2015 Elsevier Inc. All rights reserved.

outcomes, but instead initially grew because of perceived improvements in work conditions, efficiency, and theoretic gains in quality performance. Nonetheless, later multiple studies regarding internal medicine hospitalists have shown improvement in care quality for pneumonia, myocardial infarction, and hospital stay, and readmission rates.[3,4] With these quality and known workplace improvements, the utilization of hospitalists now covers a quarter of all Medicare admissions and has increased by 25% from 2009 to 2011.[5] The obstetric hospitalist movement initially developed in a similar means with limited early data, but is now progressing toward measurement of its effects on patients.

There has been a large growth in obstetric hospitalist programs over the past decade, with the recent growth rate of programs averaging 1 to 2 per month in the United States.[6] Nonetheless, there has been a paucity of clinical data on patient outcomes and this has led to a call by some to slow the growth of these programs until more data are obtained.[7] Despite this call, there exists little chance of slowdown in obstetric hospitalist program growth. Postresidency obstetric hospitalist programs have formed to fill a void in establishing special training for these providers who are becoming integral parts of the modern maternal care unit. With this workplace transformation, it has become increasingly important to document the possible changes these providers may have in the provision of intrapartum and antepartum care. As expected, data at this point are limited, as most programs are less than a decade old and many are newly developed.[6] Furthermore, unlike other disciplines, agreed-on quality measures are not generally known for maternal care, making evaluation difficult. Health care Effective Data and Information Set guidelines have been used in the past; however, these provide minimal insight on measurement of meaningful obstetric care quality. The goal of quality measurement lies in the improvement of outcomes of a healthy mother-infant unit.

Looking at the mother, maternal mortality is a rare event and maternal morbidity has only recently been given some standardized measurement options.[8] With regard to the neonate, measures indicative of true improvement in neonatal outcome are problematic to truly ascertain, as neonatal intensive care unit (NICU) admission rates, NICU length of stay, and other neonatal morbidities are affected by underlying maternal conditions and the gestational age at which they present. Furthermore, in cases with medical conditions or pregnancy-related diseases that require more intensive observation, providers increasingly send these difficult cases to a center staffed for these problems, which thus have an increased likelihood of possessing an obstetric hospitalist program. Therefore, the limited data thus far have centered on a frequently examined outcome: cesarean delivery rates.

CESAREAN DELIVERY

With more than 4 million deliveries per year in the United States, obstetric admissions are the leading cause of female hospitalization. As a measure for quality, cesarean delivery often is used as a clinical measure. Across the United States, the rate of cesarean delivery increased dramatically from 26.1% in 2002 to a stable peak of 32.8% in 2012 (**Fig. 1**).

However, as multiple clinical factors affect this outcome, the measure of unadjusted cesarean rates as a measure of quality has been considered flawed. Instead, the risk-adjusted cesarean delivery rate, primary cesarean rate, and nulliparous term singleton vertex (NTSV) cesarean delivery rate have been brought forward as more meaningful measures.[9] A measure of the NTSV rate in the entire United States is currently not available. The primary cesarean delivery rate currently exists for 38 states and

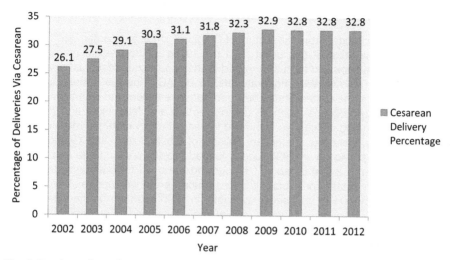

Fig. 1. Total number of cesarean deliveries in the United States from 2002 to 2012. (*Data from* National Center for Health Statistics, final natality data. Available at: www. marchofdimes.org/peristats. Accessed February 12, 2015.)

86.5% of total US births, and in 2012 stood at 21.5%. This was the first year of measurement since 2005 that this rate was less than 23.0%. However, an accepted means of determining an appropriate rate of cesarean delivery for a specific population is not easily determined due to multiple factors. Overall, the goal of prevention of the first or primary cesarean delivery for a patient has become a critical objective because of the effect on subsequent birth and the risk of cesarean delivery for subsequent gestations reaching 90%.[10]

Although many factors are responsible for primary cesarean delivery, first-stage arrest, second-stage arrest, failed induction, and nonreassuring fetal heart rate make up the vast majority of indications for laboring patients. Unfortunately, the diagnosis of arrest disorders and nonreassuring fetal heart rate status are used indiscriminately and with wide variation because of the lack of commonly applied definitions.[11] Failed induction, which also relies on physician decision-making, likewise plays a role in the variation of cesarean delivery rates. Patient attitudes and lack of appreciation regarding risks of cesarean delivery versus vaginal delivery also influence these variable risk factors. Physician work dynamics also play a nonmedical role with the increase in cesarean delivery rates. Issues of fatigue, anticipated workload, and stress contribute unnecessarily to high cesarean delivery rates and diagnoses of arrest or fetal intolerance to labor.[12,13] Awkward incentives for cesarean delivery exist due to payment systems based on fee-for-service models instead of value-based care. Current payment models providing increased pay for cesarean delivery versus vaginal birth disincentivize waiting with close observation and instead favor decisions with more rapid progress toward cesarean delivery, thereby increasing provider efficiency and reimbursement over patient outcomes. In addition, most of the payment in global obstetric fees is attributed to delivery, creating a large incentive for the provider to induce a patient to ensure birth when the obstetrician is available. Alternatively, salaried physicians have reduced incentives and, in some research, also possess lower rates of cesarean delivery.[14] Fee-for-service payment models need overhaul to aid in restoration of public confidence in physician incentives regarding decisions regarding cesarean birth.

TRIAL OF LABOR AFTER CESAREAN DELIVERY AND VAGINAL BIRTH AFTER CESAREAN

Obstetrics has changed from the dictum of Cragin,[15] "once a cesarean, always a cesarean." The evolution of this belief from the 1970s to the present has seen the pendulum swing back and forth with regard to the approach to trial of labor after cesarean delivery (TOLAC). With moderate rates of TOLAC in the 1990s, the rates of cesarean delivery in the United States dropped but were associated with an increased reporting of complications, such as uterine rupture and fetal injury and death. In 1996, McMahon and colleagues[16] showed increased major maternal morbidity with TOLAC. Shortly thereafter, American College of Obstetricians and Gynecologists (ACOG), which previously in 1994 recommended providers encourage and counsel women to undergo a trial of labor,[17] recognized the need for emergent delivery in case of sudden catastrophic complications, such as uterine rupture. They initially encouraged providers to be "readily available" in 1998 and then "immediately available" in 1999.[18,19] These changes in requirements for attendance during labor were associated with immediate and drastic decreases in TOLAC/vaginal birth after cesarean (VBAC) rates. Furthermore, although reducing primary cesarean delivery has become a major focus in decreasing overall cesarean delivery rates, the marked upswing in elective repeat cesarean delivery (ERCD) is a major contributor for the increase as well.[20] Clearly some of the declines in TOLAC have been secondary to medicolegal factors.[21] Simultaneous to this was the problem of the lack or tort reform in many states.[22] Importantly, downward trends in VBAC rates have been associated with previous exposure of a physician with complications, previous exposure to malpractice litigation, length of time in obstetric practice, and concern for risk of uterine rupture.[23]

Evaluation of the evidence regarding TOLAC clearly exhibits that successful VBAC is associated with fewer overall immediate and long-term complications. In contrast, unsuccessful VBAC leads to increased risk of maternal morbidity, including transfusion, endometritis, and uterine rupture. In comparing ERCD with TOLAC, the latter group has an apparent increase in perinatal death, but no increase in hypoxic ischemic encephalopathy or neonatal death.[24,25] However, TOLAC appears to be associated with a decreased risk of respiratory complications and hyperbilirubinemia.[26,27]

In the new era of value care, comparing cost and outcomes of TOLAC with ERCD has been necessary. Models examining cost and quality of life have shown TOLAC to save $164.2 million and gain 500 quality-adjusted life years per 100,000 women.[28] Within this same study, cost-effectiveness was found for a strategy of TOLAC over ERCD when the success rate of TOLAC was as low as 47.2%. Other studies have shown TOLAC to be more cost-effective relative to ERCD with increasing efficiency with each subsequent delivery.[29]

The Obstetrician-Gynecologist Hospitalist and Cesarean Delivery Rates

With the implementation of obstetric hospitalist programs over the past 10 years, there have been several different models of providing care. Forming these programs requires multiple staff members, financial investment, and community buy-in for success. Most programs start as nighttime or full-time coverage of a labor and delivery staffed on a rotating basis by community physicians. Some programs stay with this staffing model, but others progress to a program managed by obstetric hospitalists who are employed on a full-time basis often by the hospital or a single practice. Obstetric hospitalist programs also differ in their duties and responsibilities, with some programs covering all patients on a labor unit versus others covering drop-in patients without an assigned physician and then also assisting with cesarean deliveries, artificial rupture of membranes, and coverage of private practice patients in case of emergencies, such as sudden change in fetal status. Moreover, some units also have call responsibility for the emergency room gynecologic services (obstetric and gynecologic hospitalists). Hence, in evaluation of obstetric hospitalist programs, it is imperative to examine the type of coverage.

In the first published study of outcomes from an obstetric hospitalist program, a full-time dedicated obstetric hospitalist (laborist) program was associated with a 27% reduction in cesarean delivery when contrasted with no laborist, and 23% reduction when compared with a community physician coverage model.[30] Importantly, this study concentrated on NTSV patients and used multivariate analysis for other obstetric factors affecting cesarean delivery rates. Moreover, Iriye and colleagues[30] showed the importance of examining the type of laborist program because no reduction in cesarean delivery was exhibited when a community laborist model was used. These investigators hypothesized that this finding could be expected for several reasons. First, community physicians covering a labor unit on an occasional basis would not change their usual practice patterns to approach certain clinical scenarios, such as abnormal fetal heart rate patterns, which are not well-defined indications for cesarean delivery. Second, competitive market influences among community physicians would not allow true unencumbered collaboration in care, and hence care would still proceed under most cases similar to a no-laborist model. Third, an infrequent call schedule by a community physician as a laborist does not increase the physician's experience and comfort with their different role on labor and delivery.

Recently, a collaborative midwife/laborist model of care also showed a reduction in cesarean delivery rates. Among the NTSV patients (after adjustment for other risk factors), the traditional private practice model displayed an 86% higher risk of cesarean delivery.[31] These investigators hypothesized several reasons for the decreased cesarean delivery rates with the laborist/midwife group: (1) 24-hour in-hospital coverage of patients and (2) a group practice model with shared responsibility of the laborist/midwife patients in comparison with the private practice model. The attribution of the decreased rate of cesarean delivery in this study could be due to the laborist group, midwife provider, or both. However, a past meta-analysis displayed no difference in cesarean delivery rates with midwifery care when compared with obstetrician-provided care.[32] Hence, it would seem most likely that the laborist model coverage was responsible for the findings in the study.

The reasons for the success of these initial studies on laborist care decreasing cesarean delivery rates would seem to come from several factors. Traditional private practice care leads to conflicting demands on physician time from various sources, such as office practice, gynecologic surgery, and obstetric care. These factors may lead to decision-making processes altering care patterns.[33,34] Additionally, continued on-site coverage may lower cesarean delivery rates as well through provider comfort in waiting through problematic fetal heart rate patterns with a physician on-site. Past research showing a change of coverage to an on-site model changed physician cesarean rates and was hypothesized to occur by improved patient contact, avoidance of conflicting medical responsibility, and faster management of care.[12] Furthermore, the impact of laborist programs on cesarean delivery rates alone provide cost savings that pay for the implementation of these programs from the value they provide to the health care system.[30]

Laborist Programs and Effect on Trial of Labor After Cesarean Delivery

The inadequate rate of TOLAC in the United States has multiple consequences for medical care and diminishes health care value. Repeat cesarean delivery increases risk of placenta accreta, intraoperative surgical complications, blood loss, and transfusion, as well as escalating the risk of thromboembolism and infectious complications.[35,36] Nonetheless, enormous variation persists in the management of the patient with a previous cesarean delivery. As stated previously, low rates of TOLAC result in part from increased provider time required, malpractice risks from complications, and improper payment incentives. Obstetric hospitalist practices frequently eliminate these issues, as on-site staffing with quicker ability to respond to emergencies mitigates malpractice concerns. Additionally, many obstetric hospitalists possess a model of salaried compensation that eliminates payment incentives for cesarean delivery. Most importantly is the compliance with the immediately available standard by ACOG, which is the key critical barrier, identified to TOLAC.[37] The elimination of excessive risk resulting from these factors would appear to have a major influence in improving TOLAC rates with obstetric hospitalist care. In fact, Nijagal and colleagues[31] found dramatic reductions in elective cesarean delivery rates with an obstetric hospitalist model versus that of traditional private practice. This distinction is important, as the decrease in TOLAC does not correlate with any functional change in success rates of VBAC or patient risk patterns over the past 2 decades and appears to be due solely to provider and patient preferences.[38]

It appears likely that providers drive patients toward repeat cesarean delivery, as patients who are candidates for TOLAC seem to know very little with regard to the risks and benefits of TOLAC versus ERCD, and the mode of delivery appears to be heavily influenced by their provider preference.[39] It is difficult to determine a reason for this lack of knowledge by patients, but seems likely it is due to inappropriate counseling and directive influence by physicians. These factors would likely stem from steering patients toward repeat cesarean delivery, which requires less physician time in hospital, decreased litigation risk, and increased payment. The first 2 factors (of course) would be mitigated by use of an obstetric hospitalist program and easily explain the increased TOLAC rates in institutions using those models.

Neonatal Outcomes and Obstetric Hospitalist Coverage

Presently, the information on birth outcomes with obstetric hospitalist coverage is insufficient and more research is required.[7] Throughout the United States, many community hospitals operate without full-time obstetric coverage of patients on labor and delivery, with many decisions made and interventions performed by nursing staff. In rural areas, physician shortages may necessitate this care model without 24-hour on-site coverage to allow basic obstetric services when there is no other alternative. Although there are conflicting data, timing of delivery of cases characterized by obstetric emergencies remains critical to enhance neonatal outcomes. Within the United States, more than one-third of all emergent deliveries occur outside of the ACOG-recommended 30-minute delivery interval.[40] However, examining infants delivered within the 30-minute time period there was higher apparent compromise with more umbilical artery pH less than 7 and elevated rates of delivery room intubation. Most likely this reflects the need for true emergent delivery secondary to the underlying cause of the event and indicates a need in some scenarios for delivery with further reduction of decision to delivery time rather than the arbitrary time of 30 minutes. For example, Chauhan and colleagues[41] found a higher level of adverse neonatal outcome with a decision to incision interval of more than 30 minutes. Hence, although these 2 studies differ, it is hard to argue that in a true obstetric emergency, an avoidable delay in intervention would lead to improved neonatal outcomes.

A key concept of obstetric hospitalist coverage is the provision of 24-hour in-house call to provide improved neonatal and maternal outcomes. Goffman and colleagues,[42] with a program of institution of obstetric best practices, including fetal heart monitoring training, educational intervention, simulation, enhanced documentation, and 24-hour enhanced call, showed a 42% reduction in maternal and neonatal adverse events. In-hospital coverage would reasonably lead to decreased response time from off-site call schemes, providing better care and possible better outcomes in cases such as cord prolapse, fetal bradycardia, uterine rupture, and abruption. Additional possible benefits of full-time obstetric hospitalists in these scenarios may also result from more experience, lack of sleep deprivation, and improved communication with nursing staff. However, further studies are needed to corroborate these theoretic advantages.

SUMMARY

Obstetric hospitalist programs are rapidly increasing in the United States as a means to provide 24-hour labor coverage while simultaneously striving to improve patient safety, reduce malpractice liability risk, and decrease physician burnout. The US medical system currently is moving toward a system of value-based care, with a more focused look on maternal and infant outcomes. Specific factors to be measured with regard to patient quality have not been universally determined. Cesarean delivery rates have been examined as a possible metric because of effects on maternal and infant health, as well as effects on medical costs. Obstetric hospitalists, especially those professionals functioning as full-time hospitalist providers, appear to have a significant impact on reducing cesarean delivery rates. In addition, TOLAC/VBAC rates appear to improve in hospitals with obstetric hospitalist programs. The examination of cesarean delivery rates and other quality metrics within these programs deserves further investigation, but preliminary evidence shows promising effects on decreasing cesarean delivery.

REFERENCES

1. Wachter RM, Goldman L. The emerging role of "hospitalists" in the American health care system. N Engl J Med 1996;335:514–7.
2. Weinstein L. The laborist: a new focus of practice for the obstetrician. Am J Obstet Gynecol 2003;188:310–2.
3. Jungerwirth R, Wheeler SB, Paul JE. Association of hospitalist presence and hospital-level outcome measures among Medicare patients. J Hosp Med 2014; 9:1–6.
4. Vasilevkis EE, Knebel RJ, Dudley RA, et al. Cross sectional analysis of hospitalist prevalence and quality of care in California. J Hosp Med 2010;5:200–7.
5. Welch WP, Stearns SC, Cuellar AE, et al. Use of hospitalists by Medicare beneficiaries: a national picture. Medicare Medicaid Res Rev 2014;4:E1–8.
6. Olson R, Garite TJ, Fishman A, et al. Obstetrician/gynecologist hospitalists: can we improve safety and outcomes for patients and hospitals and improve lifestyle for physicians? Am J Obstet Gynecol 2012;8:81–6.
7. Srinivas SK, Lorch SA. The laborist model of obstetric care: we need more evidence. Am J Obstet Gynecol 2012;7:30–5.
8. Grobman WA, Bailit JL, Rice MM, et al. Frequency of and factors associated with severe maternal morbidity. Obstet Gynecol 2014;4:804–10.
9. Bailit JL. Measuring the quality of inpatient obstetrical care. Obstet Gynecol Surv 2007;3:207–13.
10. Spong CY, Berghella V, Wenstrom KD, et al. Preventing the first cesarean delivery: summary of a joint Eunice Kennedy Shriver National Institute of Child Health

and Human Development, Society for Maternal-Fetal Medicine, and American College of Obstetricians and Gynecologists workshop. Obstet Gynecol 2012; 120:1181–93.

11. Brennan DJ, Robson MS, Murphy M, et al. Comparative analysis of international cesarean delivery rates using 10-group classification identifies significant variation in spontaneous labor. Am J Obstet Gynecol 2009;201(3):308.e1–8.

12. Klasko SK, Cummings RV, Balducci J, et al. The impact of mandated in-hospital coverage on primary cesarean delivery rates in a large non-university teaching hospital. Am J Obstet Gynecol 1995;172(2 Pt 1):637–42.

13. Spetz J, Smith MW, Ennis SF. Physician incentives and the timing of cesarean sections: evidence from California. Med Care 2001;39:536–50.

14. Macones GA, Hankins GD, Spong CY, et al. The 2008 National Institute of Child Health and Human Development workshop report on electronic fetal monitoring: update on definitions, interpretation, and research guidelines. Obstet Gynecol 2008;112:661–6.

15. Cragin EB. Conservatism in obstetrics. NY Med J 1916;104:1–3.

16. McMahon MJ, Luther ER, Bowes WA, et al. Comparison of trial of labor with an elective second cesarean section. N Engl J Med 1996;335:689–95.

17. American College of Obstetricians and Gynecologists. Vaginal delivery after previous cesarean birth. Washington, DC: ACOG; 1994. Committee opinion No. 143.

18. American College of Obstetricians and Gynecologists. Vaginal delivery after previous cesarean delivery. Washington, DC: ACOG; 1998. Practice Bulletin Number 2.

19. American College of Obstetricians and Gynecologists. Vaginal delivery after previous cesarean section. Washington, DC: ACOG; 1999. Practice Bulletin Number 5.

20. Barber EL, Lundsberg LS, Belanger K, et al. Indications contributing to the increasing cesarean delivery rate. Obstet Gynecol 2011;118:29–38.

21. Xu X, Siefert KA, Jacobson PD, et al. The effects of medical liability on obstetrical care supply in Michigan. Am J Obstet Gynecol 2008;198:e1–9.

22. Yang TY, Mello MM, Subramanian SV, et al. Relationship between malpractice litigation pressure and rates of cesarean section and vaginal birth after cesarean section. Med Care 2009;47:234–42.

23. Wells ED. Vaginal birth after cesarean delivery: views from the private practitioner. Semin Perinatol 2010;34:345–50.

24. Landon MB, Hauth JC, Leveno KJ, et al. Maternal and perinatal outcomes associated with a trial of labor after prior cesarean delivery. National Institute of Child Health and Human Development maternal-fetal medicine units network. N Engl J Med 2004;351:2581–9.

25. Smith GC, Pell JP, Cameron AD, et al. Risk of perinatal death associated with labor after previous cesarean delivery in uncomplicated term pregnancies. JAMA 2002;287:2684–90.

26. Signore C, Hemachandra A, Klebanoff M. Neonatal mortality and morbidity after elective cesarean delivery versus routine expectant management: a decision analysis. Semin Perinatol 2006;30:288–95.

27. Hook B, Kiwi R, Amini SB, et al. Neonatal morbidity after elective repeat cesarean section and trial of labor. Pediatrics 1997;100:348–53.

28. Gilbert SA, Grobman WA, Landon MB, et al. Lifetime cost-effectiveness of trial of labor after cesarean in the United States. Value Health 2013;16(6):953–64.

29. Wymer KM, Shi Y-CT, Plunkett BA. The cost-effectiveness of a trial of labor accrues with multiple subsequent vaginal deliveries. Am J Obstet Gynecol 2014; 211:56.e1–12.

30. Iriye BK, Huang WH, Condon J, et al. Implementation of a laborist program and evaluation of the effect upon cesarean delivery. Am J Obstet Gynecol 2013;209: 251.e1–6.

31. Nijagal MA, Kuppermann M, Nakagawa S, et al. Two practice models in one labor and delivery unit: association with cesarean delivery rates. Am J Obstet Gynecol 2014;212:1.e1–8.

32. Hatem M, Sandall J, Devane D, et al. Midwife-led versus other models of care for childbearing women. Cochrane Database Syst Rev 2008;(4):CD004667.

33. Bailit J. Impact of non-clinical factors on primary cesarean deliveries. Semin Perinatol 2012;36:395–8.

34. Poma PA. Effect of departmental policies on cesarean delivery rates: a community hospital experience. Obstet Gynecol 1998;91:1013–8.

35. Zia S, Rafique M. Intra-operative complications increase with successive number of cesarean sections: myth or fact? Obstet Gynecol Sci 2014;57(3):187–92.

36. Gasim T, Al Jama FE, Rahman MS, et al. Multiple repeat cesarean sections: operative difficulties, maternal complications and outcome. J Reprod Med 2013; 58(7–8):312–8.

37. Cottrell EKB, Wasson N, Wagner J, et al. Vaginal birth after Cesarean: developing and prioritizing a future research agenda. Future research needs Paper No. 15. (Prepared by the Oregon evidence-based practice center under contract No. 290-2007-10057-I.) AHRQ Publication No. 12-EHC072-EF. Rockville (MD): Agency for Healthcare Research and Quality; 2012 (addendum August 2012).

38. Grobman WA, Lai Y, Landon MB, et al. The change in the rate of vaginal birth after caesarean section. Paediatr Perinat Epidemiol 2011;25(1):37–43.

39. Ernstein SN, Matalon-Grazi S, Rosenn BM. Trial of labor versus repeat cesarean: are patients making an informed decision? Am J Obstet Gynecol 2012;207: 204.e1–6.

40. Bloom SL, Leveno KJ, Spong CY, et al. Decision to incision times and maternal and infant outcomes. Obstet Gynecol 2006;108(1):6–11.

41. Chauhan SP, Roach H, Naef RW II, et al. Cesarean section for suspected fetal distress. Does the decision–incision time make a difference? J Reprod Med 1997;42:347–52.

42. Goffman D, Broadman M, Arnold AJ, et al. Improved obstetric safety through programmatic collaboration. J Healthc Risk Manag 2014;33(3):14–22.

Potential Impact of Obstetrics and Gynecology Hospitalists on Safety of Obstetric Care

CrossMark

Sindhu K. Srinivas, MD, MSCE

KEYWORDS

- Hospitalist • Pregnancy • Safety • OBGYN hospitalist • Infant mortality
- Maternal mortality

KEY POINTS

- Obstetrics and gynecology (OBGYN) hospitalists are growing nationally, with the impetus largely being improved patient safety.
- It is plausible that OBGYN hospitalists could improve outcomes, both overall and in the setting of unpredictable obstetric emergencies.
- More literature is desperately needed to evaluate the impact of OBGYN hospitalists on patient safety and outcomes.
- This literature would have significant policy implications for obstetric care delivery nationally and financing of OBGYN prenatal and delivery care.

INTRODUCTION

More than 4 million women give birth annually in the United States, making child birth one of the most common reasons for hospital care[1] and amplifying the significance of changes in complications. Although there is almost universal agreement on the need for improved safety, care delivery models to achieve this goal of safer care are evolving.

The obstetrics and gynecology (OBGYN) hospitalist is a relatively recent focus within obstetrics and gynecology. The need for continual surveillance of patients during labor and delivery, not needed in most medicine hospitalist services, and the acute nature of most obstetric emergencies offer a unique mechanism for improving safety and outcomes with the OBGYN hospitalist model that differs from the hospitalist

Department of Obstetrics and Gynecology, Perelman School of Medicine, University of Pennsylvania, 3400 Spruce Street, 5 Dulles, Philadelphia, PA 19104, USA
E-mail address: ssrinivas@obgyn.upenn.edu

Obstet Gynecol Clin N Am 42 (2015) 487–491
http://dx.doi.org/10.1016/j.ogc.2015.05.007
0889-8545/15/$ – see front matter © 2015 Elsevier Inc. All rights reserved.

obgyn.theclinics.com

model of medicine. The OBGYN hospitalist is traditionally viewed as a trained OBGYN who is hired primarily to work on labor and delivery. In this capacity, OBGYN hospitalists are touted as having an expanded knowledge base on labor and delivery, focused on safety and quality initiatives and patient satisfaction and the patient experience on labor and delivery. Continuous coverage on labor and delivery may also be achieved by pooling provider staff and changing traditional coverage models of individual practices to more of a shift-based labor and delivery coverage. Further, there are many hybrids of both OBGYN hospitalists covering labor and delivery at nighttime or in conjunction with private practice or academic practice providers to create a model of continuous coverage. Regardless of the model of implementation, hospitals often cite improved patient safety implications as the primary driver for moving to OBGYN hospitalists in their obstetric care delivery model.[2]

Although there is no literature to date specifically demonstrating improved safety with OBGYN hospitalists, several circumstantial pieces of evidence support the potential critical role of the OBGYN hospitalists/OBGYN hospitalist model in improving the safety of labor and delivery units.

THE PROBLEM OF MATERNAL MORTALITY

Ninety-nine percent of all births occur in a hospital. Almost 92% of these births are performed by physicians. Midwife births account for approximately 8% of all births, and 93% of midwife-staffed births occur in a hospital setting.[3] With the exception of unsafe pregnancy terminations, most maternal deaths and two-thirds of infant deaths occur between the onset of labor and 28 days post partum.[4,5] Although there was a dramatic decline in maternal mortality in the United States in the twentieth century, there has been little further reduction in the last 20 years. Specifically, maternal mortality in the United States is 1 per 4800 deliveries; the United States ranks 41st in the world for this health indicator behind most industrialized countries.[6] In the United States, the major causes of maternal mortality include preeclampsia, hemorrhage, embolism, infection, and complications from preexisting medical conditions. Three major delays are responsible for most maternal mortality: (1) a delay in a decision to seek care, (2) a delay in transportation to a health care facility, and (3) a delay in receiving care at a health care facility.[7] Timely access to emergency obstetric services significantly reduces the number of maternal deaths.[8] However, barriers to care, including lack of adequate facilities, insufficient transportation, and inadequate supply of health care providers, have resulted in little improvement in maternal mortality in developing nations. According to the World Health Organization, to reduce the maternal mortality ratio by three-quarters before 2015, improving health care for women and providing universal access to reproductive health services is essential. Among these services is the provision of high-quality pregnancy and delivery care, including emergency obstetric care. Specifically, when obstetric emergencies arise during pregnancy and delivery, the importance of recognizing danger signs and seeking care quickly is critical.[9]

INFANT MORTALITY

In addition to maternal mortality, another important national health indicator is infant mortality rate. This measure is considered one of the most important health indicators of a nation because it is thought to be an indicator of a variety of other factors such as maternal health and quality of care. Since 2000 the infant mortality rate has not declined in the United States. As of 2004, the infant mortality ranking is 29th, less than most other comparable nations.[10] The major causes of these deaths include infection, birth asphyxia, birth injuries, preterm births, and birth defects.[6] Additionally, fetal death (defined as the death of fetuses before birth) is another important indicator of perinatal health, and this rate has remained relatively stagnant over the last 20 years. These deaths are largely caused by obstetric or maternal complications. Intrapartum fetal deaths can also occur, although they occur more often in developing nations where births are often not attended by a skilled attendant. A recent study reported a 0.6 per 1000 rate of intrapartum stillbirth largely caused by chorioamnionitis, cord prolapse, and abruptio placenta.[11] Intrapartum deaths are thought to result from sub-optimal management of labor and delivery whereby timely recognition and management may have prevented the death from occurring.[6,12–14]

TIMELINESS OF DELIVERY IN EMERGENT SITUATIONS

Recognizing the importance of timely recognition and response to emergent situations on improving maternal and neonatal outcomes, the American College of Obstetricians and Gynecologists' (ACOG) guidelines recommend that all hospitals have the "capability of performing a cesarean delivery within 30 minutes of the decision to operate" but "not all indications for a cesarean delivery will require a 30 minute response time."[15,16] Often, as in the case of abruptio placenta or cord prolapse, the time interval to delivery should be less than 30 minutes. The early recognition of many peripartum events, including infection, hemorrhage, and obstructed labor, can result in a reduction in maternal and infant mortality during labor, delivery, and neonatal periods.[6] Therefore, it is plausible that OBGYN hospitalists, with the premise of a continuous, well-rested, trained staff presence on labor and delivery, may improve maternal and neonatal outcomes.

PREVENTABLE PERINATAL OUTCOMES WITH CLOSE MONITORING AND INTERVENTION

Although many births occur without complication, the gravity of complications and the inability to predict which pregnancies they will affect creates the need for clinical vigilance. Several pregnancy-related disorders, labor complications, and use of medications require constant attention to avoid adverse outcomes.

Hemorrhage

Hemorrhage and hypertension are 2 major causes of mortality and intensive care unit admissions from obstetric services.[17] Obstetric hemorrhage is the leading cause of both maternal mortality and severe morbidity worldwide and contributes to approximately 24% of all maternal deaths.[4] If unrecognized and uncontrolled, hemorrhage can lead to shock and death in a short period of time. Immediate hemorrhage is often caused by uterine atony and requires early recognition, assessment, and intervention with manual evacuation of retained products, bimanual massage, and uterotonic medication administration.[18] Recent data from Australia and the United States demonstrated an increase in postpartum hemorrhage in blood product transfusion from 1999 to 2004.[19,20] Additionally, newly implemented patient safety bundles addressing the recognition and coordinated management of obstetric hemorrhage has demonstrated improved maternal patient safety and outcomes, specifically demonstrating a reduction in transfusion and need for peripartum hysterectomy.[21]

Use of Oxytocin

Oxytocin is a widely used medication in labor augmentation and is described as the drug most associated with preventable adverse events in childbirth.[22] Although its use is sometimes necessary to augment labor, its use can also result in detrimental effects through doses causing excess uterine activity. The highly variable effects from patient to patient make surveillance of its use critical in preventing uterine overactivity.[22]

THE ROLE OF THE OBSTETRICS AND GYNECOLOGY HOSPITALIST IN PATIENT SAFETY

In 2010, The American Congress of Obstetricians and Gynecologists issued a committee opinion on OBGYN hospitalists that acknowledged their potential to solve or improve many of the problems and concerns that are addressed in this article, stating that it "supports the continued development of the OBGYN hospitalist model as one potential approach to achieving increased professional and patient satisfaction while maintaining safe and effective care across delivery settings."[23] At the inaugural meeting of the Society of Obstetrician/Gynecologist Hospitalist in October 2011, the ACOG District VIII chair, Joshua Kopelman, gave credence to OBGYN hospitalists, stating: "ACOG recognizes this is the new paradigm of care" and that "OB/GYN hospitalists in this country are the wave of the future. There's no question about it."[23]

OBGYN hospitalists have the potential ability to impact patient safety in several ways, including as seasoned clinicians taking on the role of experts in obstetric emergencies, as leaders in the daily operations of labor and delivery units, as educators in the training of house staff, and as patient safety officers and leaders in the development and implementers of important safety and quality initiatives.

SUMMARY/DISCUSSION

Although it is plausible for OBGYN hospitalists to impact patient safety, there is wide variation in the models of OBGYN hospitalist utilization. Variations exist among practicing OBGYN hospitalists because of individual, institutional, and societal/contextual differences. Some have proposed better defining the model by establishing a fellowship in inpatient-obstetrics/OBGYN hospitalist care providing the structure to training in providing obstetric care that is given to other OBGYN subspecialties.[24] Although this may be the wave of the future in OBGYN, one thing is clear: OBGYN hospitalist programs are rapidly being adopted in numerous hospitals across the country.[25] In order for these programs to have the largest impact on patient safety and maternal and neonatal outcomes, a few things need to occur. First, we need to implement flexible models that are most responsive to the needs of individual hospitals. Second, we need to create tools to effectively study the impact of different OBGYN hospitalist models on patient safety and perinatal outcomes in order to develop an improved evidence base for different obstetric care delivery models. Third, we need to address the payment and reimbursement structure of obstetric and labor and delivery care to incentivize safe practice.

REFERENCES

1. National Center for Health Statistics. Centers for Disease Control. 2008.
2. Jesus A, Caldwell D, Srinivas SK. Why hospitals adopt the laborist model of obstetric care: a qualitative analysis. J Women's Health Gynecol, in press.
3. Martin J, Hamilton B. Births: final data for 2006. Natl Vital Stat Rep 2009;57(7).
4. World Health Organization (WHO). Reduction of maternal mortality: a joint WHO/UNFPA/World Bank Statement. Geneva: WHO; 1999.
5. Li XF, Fortney JA, Kotelchuck M, et al. The postpartum period: the key to maternal mortality. Int J Gynaecol Obstet 1996;54(1):1–10.

6. Bale JR, Stoll BJ, Lucas AO. Improving birth outcomes: meeting the challenge in the developing world. Institute of Medicine of the National Academies. Washington, DC: The National Academies Press; 2003.

7. Safe motherhood fact sheet. Reproductive Health Response in Conflict Consortium 2008.

8. Maternal mortality update: a focus on emergency obstetric care. New York: United Nations Population Fund; 2002.

9. Maternal mortality ratio falling too slowly to meet goal World Health Organization. 2007.

10. MacDorman MF, Matthews TJ. Recent trends in infant mortality in the United States. NCHS Data Brief 2008;(9):1–8.

11. Getahun D, Ananth CV, Kinzler WL. Risk factors for antepartum and intrapartum stillbirth. Am J Obstet Gynecol 2007;196(6):499–507.

12. Kiely JL, Paneth N, Susser M. Fetal death during labor: an epidemiologic indicator of level of obstetric care. Am J Obstet Gynecol 1985;153(7):721–7.

13. Sheiner E, Hallak M, Shoham-Vardi I, et al. Determining risk factors for intrapartum fetal death. J Reprod Med 2000;45(5):419–24.

14. Stewart JH, Andrews J, Cartlidge PH. Numbers of deaths related to intrapartum asphyxia and timing of birth in all Wales perinatal survey, 1993-5. BMJ 1998; 316(7132):657–60.

15. Gabbe SG, Niebyl JR, Simpson JL. Obstetrics normal and problem pregnancies. 5th Edition. Philadelphia: Churchhill Livingstonstone Elsevier; 2007.

16. Lucas DN, Yentis SM, Kinsella SM, et al. Urgency of caesarean section: a new classification. J R Soc Med 2000;93(7):346–50.

17. American College of Obstetricians and Gynecologists. ACOG practice bulletin number 100: critical care in pregnancy. Obstet Gynecol 2009;113(2):443–50.

18. ACOG practice bulletin number 76: postpartum hemorrhage. 2006.

19. Rochelson B. D-O-G years. Obstet Gynecol 2003;101(5 Pt 1):1008.

20. Srinivas SK, Epstein AJ, Nicholson S, et al. Improvements in US maternal obstetrical outcomes from 1992 to 2006. Med Care 2010;48(5):487–93.

21. Shields LE, Wiesner S, Fulton J, et al. Comprehensive maternal hemorrhage protocols reduce the use of blood products and improve patient safety. Am J Obstet Gynecol 2015;212(3):272–80.

22. Clark SL, Simpson KR, Knox GE, et al. Oxytocin: new perspectives on an old drug. Am J Obstet Gynecol 2009;200(1):35.e1–6.

23. Committee opinion no. 459: the obstetric-gynecologic hospitalist. Obstet Gynecol 2010;116(1):237–9.

24. Atallah F. What is a laborist? Am J Obstet Gynecol 2013;208(5):418.

25. Olson R, Garite TJ, Fishman A, et al. Obstetrician/gynecologist hospitalists: can we improve safety and outcomes for patients and hospitals and improve lifestyle for physicians? Am J Obstet Gynecol 2012;207(2):81–6.

Sleep Deprivation

Robert M. Abrams, MD

KEYWORDS

- Sleep deprivation • Sleep • Physician fatigue • Residency program • Hospitalist
- Fatigue management • Pregnancy

KEY POINTS

- Sleep deprivation occurs when inadequate sleep leads to decreased performance, inadequate alertness, and deterioration in health.
- Energy conservation, restoration, and information processing are different theories as to why humans need sleep.
- Sleep deprivation has many deleterious effects, including increased risk for stroke, obesity, diabetes, cancer, permanent cognitive deficits, osteoporosis, cardiovascular disease, and mortality.
- During pregnancy, sleep deprivation increases the risk for preeclampsia, gestational diabetes, intrauterine growth restriction, and need for cesarean delivery.
- Physicians who work recurrent 24-hour shifts make 36% more medical errors, double their risk for motor vehicle crash when driving home, have less empathy for patients, and have an increase in family and marital stress.
- Hospitalist programs are structured to enhance patient safety, decrease malpractice risk, and improve the physician's quality of life.

INTRODUCTION

Sleep deprivation occurs when inadequate sleep leads to decreased performance, inadequate alertness, and deterioration in health. Sleep deprivation is extremely common, with 20% of the adult population reported to be sleep deprived. Inadequate sleep is due to either decreased quantity or impaired quality of sleep. Typically, a decrease in quantity of sleep occurs over multiple nights. If chronic, loss of sleep results in a sleep debt, which cannot be recovered.[1] Although the amount of sleep required varies from person to person, on average, 7 to 8 hours of sleep are needed per night to function without impairment. Even if a person sleeps more than 8 hours nightly, sleep deprivation may still occur if the quality of this sleep is poor. Sleep quality

Division of Maternal Fetal Medicine, Department of Obstetrics and Gynecology, Southern Illinois University School of Medicine, 415 North Ninth Street, 6W100, PO Box 19640, Springfield, IL 62794, USA
E-mail address: rabrams@siumed.edu

Obstet Gynecol Clin N Am 42 (2015) 493–506
http://dx.doi.org/10.1016/j.ogc.2015.05.013
0889-8545/15/$ – see front matter © 2015 Elsevier Inc. All rights reserved.

obgyn.theclinics.com

is determined by the number of arousals, or awakenings from sleep, during the night. Five or more arousals can lead to daytime sleepiness.[2]

Pregnant women and obstetrician-gynecologists (OB/GYNs) themselves are affected by sleep deprivation, and signs and symptoms of this disorder must be recognized to optimize the care of our patients as well as ourselves.

WHY DO HUMANS SLEEP?

Sleep is typically defined as a state of reduced responsiveness, motor activity, and metabolism. It is distinguished from coma or anesthesia by its rapid reversibility. Despite the fact that humans spend one-third of their life sleeping, why sleep is needed remains poorly understood. It is theorized that sleep fulfills some universal virtual function that is yet unknown.[3]

Sleep can be categorized into 2 alternating cycles: rapid eye movement (REM) sleep and non-REM (NREM) sleep. Each night, 5 cycles of sleep typically occur. Most adults begin sleep from the drowsy state (NREM). NREM is divided into 3 substages: stage N1, stage N2, and stage N3 (**Fig. 1, Table 1**).

- Stage N1: Transition from wakefulness to sleep. Eye movements are slow and rolling. This stage is the lightest stage of sleep. If one awakens from stage N1 sleep, the individual may not perceive that he or she was ever asleep.[4]
- Stage N2: This stage comprises the greatest percentage of total sleep time (50% of the night). Electroencephalography (EEG) frequency slows, thus leading to deeper sleep.
- Stage N3: Deep sleep. This stage accounts for 10% to 20% of sleep time. EEG frequency is at its slowest during this stage. It is most difficult to awaken during this stage of sleep.
- REM sleep: REM sleep may also be called stage R. An EEG during REM sleep resembles that of an active, awake person. Because of the similarity to wakefulness, REM sleep is also called paradoxic sleep.[5] It is during REM sleep that vivid dreaming occurs. Only 20% of sleeping time is in REM stage, and the function of this stage is unclear.[2]

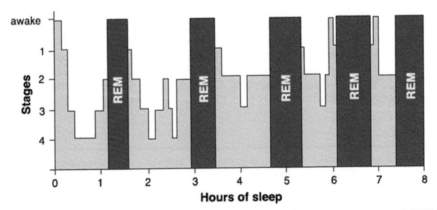

Fig. 1. Typical hypnogram from a young, healthy adult. Light-gray areas represent NREM sleep. (*From* Biological Sciences Curriculum Study. Sleep, sleep disorders, and biological rhythms. Bethesda (MD): National Institutes of Health; 2003. NIH publication no. 04-4989.)

Table 1
Comparison of physiologic changes during NREM and REM sleep

Physiologic Process	During NREM	During REM
Brain activity	Decreases from wakefulness	Increases in motor and sensory areas, whereas other areas are similar to NREM
Heart rate	Slows from wakefulness	Increases and varies compared with NREM
Blood pressure	Decreases from wakefulness	Increases (up to 30%) and varies from NREM
Blood flow to brain	Does not change from wakefulness in most regions	Increases by 50% to 200% from NREM, depending on brain region
Respiration	Decreases from wakefulness	Increases and varies from NREM, but may show brief stoppages (apnea); coughing suppressed
Airway resistance	Increases from wakefulness	Increases and varies from wakefulness
Body temperature	Is regulated at lower set point than wakefulness; shivering initiated at lower temperature than during wakefulness	Is not regulated; no shivering or sweating; temperature drifts toward that of the local environment
Sexual arousal	Occurs infrequently	Increases from NREM (in both men and women)

From Biological Sciences Curriculum Study. Sleep, sleep disorders, and biological rhythms. Bethesda (MD): National Institutes of Health; 2003. NIH publication no. 04-4989.

There are multiple theories as to why humans need sleep:

- Energy conservation theory: From an evolutionary perspective, if food was scarce, then this state of lowered caloric needs would promote survival.
- Restorative theory: This theory implies that the body rejuvenates and repairs during sleep. Sleep reverses damage that occurs in waking, including oxidative stress, depletion of energy stores, death of neurons in the hippocampus, and downregulation of receptors.
- Information processing theory: This theory argues that sleep promotes learning and storage of memories by returning saturated learning circuits back to baseline levels.[6]

SLEEP DEPRIVATION

The first study on sleep deprivation was published more than 100 years ago.[7] Since then, the meaning of sleep, as well as the ramifications of being sleep deprived, have been extensively studied.

Causes of sleep deprivation are as follows[8]:

- Voluntary behavior. These are people who engage in voluntary behaviors that lead to unintentional chronic sleep deprivation. Prevalent examples of voluntary behavior are staying up late each evening to watch television or surf the Internet. There must be a pattern of restricted sleep that is present almost daily for at least 3 months.
- Personal obligations. For example, a person may lose significant sleep while providing care for an ill relative.

- ○ Work hours. Some occupations can produce sleep deprivation. Obviously, OB/GYNs are included in this category.
- ○ Medical problems. Certain medical conditions, such as sleep apnea, may not allow uninterrupted sleep. The prevalence of sleep apnea is dramatically increasing due to an increase in chronic diseases such as hypertension and obesity. At present, 42 million American adults have sleep apnea.[9]

Sleep deprivation has many deleterious effects[10]:

- ○ Increased risk for stroke. Adults who sleep fewer than 6 hours per night have a 4-fold elevated risk of stroke
- ○ Obesity due to increased production of ghrelin and limited production of leptin
- ○ Elevated risk of diabetes due to an increase in insulin resistance
- ○ Permanent cognitive deficits
- ○ Mental status changes resembling depression or anxiety
- ○ Quality of life is reported as worse.
- ○ Osteoporosis
- ○ Increased risk for colorectal and breast cancer
- ○ A 48% higher risk of developing cardiovascular disease
- ○ Increase in mortality. During a 14-year study period, men who slept less than 6 hours per night were 4 times more likely to die during the study period

As one ages, sleep deprivation worsens because of an increase in sleep disorders and decreased quality of sleep. After age 45 years, deep stage 3 and 4 levels are lessened, which makes it more difficult for older physicians to function after a sleepless night on call when compared with their younger colleagues.[11] Along with cognitive impairment seen in sleep-deprived physicians, there are considerable emotional effects. Physicians who lack quality sleep have a significant increase in depression, lack of empathy toward patients, marital discord, and suicide.[12]

Sleep deprivation seems to be worsening in our society, as the prevalence of short sleep (<6 hours per night) increased from 7.6% in 1975 to 9.3% in 2006.[13] Sleepiness-related incidents cost billions of dollars annually.[14] Several disasters in recent history have been attributed to sleep deprivation, including the Exxon Valdez oil spill, 3 Mile Island, and the space shuttle disaster.[15] In addition, 25% of all train accidents in the past 5 years were attributed directly to fatigue.[16] Because these significant disasters may have been prevented with proper sleep hygiene, the transportation industry and others enacted strict regulations regarding work and rest time. For example, the US Code of Federal Regulations requirements[17] include the following:

- Pilots: Domestic pilots may not fly more than 30 hours per week, 100 hours per month, or 1000 hours per year.
- Truck drivers: Commercial truck drivers must drive no more than 10 hours daily and 60 hours per week. After a 10-hour day, truckers must have 8 consecutive hours off.
- Marine operators: Those in charge of marine vessel navigation must have 10 hours of rest in 24 hours.

Although many medical errors and malpractice cases have been linked to physician fatigue, the US government has not created work and rest time regulations for physicians as it has for the previously mentioned occupations.

CAN SLEEP DEPRIVATION BE CURED?

To combat sleep deprivation, there have been many advisements from varying organizations. Sleeping in for several days in a row may help one feel better rested. If

nightly sleep cannot be extended, short 15 to 20 minute naps during the day may lead to heightened alertness. Other ways to mitigate fatigue include regular physical activity, bright light, caffeine, or prescription analeptics.[18] However, to cure sleep deprivation, sleep habits must be permanently restructured. An individual must make lifestyle changes to obtain adequate and good-quality sleep.

SLEEP DEPRIVATION IN THE AGE OF ELECTRONICS

Proper sleep hygiene is important in optimizing sleep and minimizing sleep deficit. The bedroom should only be used for sleep. Televisions, personal electronic devices, and other blue-light distractions should be removed from the bedroom. A 2014 poll by the National Sleep Foundation offered a glimpse into just how pervasive electronics have become in American bedrooms. About 90% of adults reported having at least 1 electronic device in their bedroom, and many admitted to having multiple devices, such as televisions, laptops, and tablets.[19] Furthermore, 26% of respondents said that they sent or read text messages, e-mails, or other electronic communications after they had initially gone to sleep at least once in the week preceding the survey.

Unplugging before going to bed proves to be a difficult task. However, it is essential that electronic devices do not accompany the individual into the bedroom. There are significant scientific data correlating light with promoting wakefulness. Photoreceptors in the retina sense light and dark, which allows the brain to align the circadian rhythm to the external day-night cycle. This signaling of light and dark enables one to be alert in the morning and fall asleep at the appropriate time at night. Small electronic devices emit enough light to miscue the brain and promote wakefulness at night, which over time permanently alters the circadian rhythm and leads to chronic sleep deprivation.[20]

A study by Chang and colleagues[21] evaluated the effects of using electronic devices in the hours before bedtime. They concluded that using light-emitting electronic devices before bedtime contributes to sleep deprivation by the following mechanisms:

- Prolongs the time it takes to fall asleep
- Delays the circadian clock
- Suppresses levels of melatonin, the sleep-promoting hormone
- Reduces the amount, and delays the timing of, REM sleep
- Reduces alertness the following morning
- Increases alertness immediately before bedtime, which leads to delayed bedtime

SLEEP DEPRIVATION IN PREGNANCY

Sleep disturbance of any kind during pregnancy negatively affects obstetric outcomes. Compared with the general population in which 67% of women report sleeps problems at least a few nights a week, 84% of pregnant women have sleep disturbances.[22] Total sleep time among pregnant women is 35.8 minutes shorter than their nonpregnant counterparts.[23]

Changes in sleep architecture are mainly due to more frequent stage changes and decrease in REM sleep, likely due to increased progesterone levels.[24] As pregnancy progresses, sleep patterns become consistent with an insomnia pattern due to REM sleep suppression and increasing wake time. This pattern ultimately results in sleep deprivation, which worsens pregnancy outcomes.[25]

In a questionnaire-based study of pregnant resident physicians, when compared with spouses of male colleagues, there was an increased risk of preterm labor (11% vs 6%), preterm delivery (9.8% vs 3.5%), and preeclampsia (8.8% vs 3.5%).[26] Although sleep was not directly evaluated, the hours worked weekly were almost doubled in the pregnant resident physicians. The study concluded that sleep deprivation played a role in the increased obstetric complications seen in the pregnant residents.

A study by Louis and colleagues[27] concluded that obstructive sleep apnea (OSA) increases the risk for hypertensive disorders of pregnancy (gestational hypertension and preeclampsia). Sleep deprivation is a risk factor for OSA, thus increasing the probability of hypertensive complications. Other complications of short sleep duration during pregnancy include gestational diabetes,[28] increased risk for cesarean delivery,[29] and intrauterine growth restriction. The hypothesis associating sleep deprivation with adverse obstetric outcomes is that inflammatory pathways, specifically interleukin (IL)-6 levels, are stimulated when a pregnant woman is sleep deprived. Increased circulating IL-6 levels have been associated with the aforementioned outcomes, especially preeclampsia.[30]

Because of the proven risks of sleep deprivation in pregnancy, the importance of proper rest and sleep during pregnancy is often discussed at a woman's initial prenatal visit by her obstetrician. However, it is not uncommon for that same OB/GYN to work greater than 100 hours per week, thus leading to marked fatigue and sleep deprivation. By not following our own recommendations of proper sleep hygiene and setting an example, it is more difficult for patients to heed our advice.

EVOLUTION OF WORK RESTRICTIONS FOR RESIDENCY PROGRAMS

The first residency program in 1889 was at Johns Hopkins Hospital under the direction of Sir William Osler. Newly graduated medical students underwent intense medical training, whereby they lived at the hospital an entire year, thus coining the term resident. During the next century, residency programs continued to be associated with intense training. Oftentimes, residents worked more than 48 hours consecutively. It was not until 1971, when a study showed significantly more errors in electrocardiogram interpretation by postcall residents compared with their rested colleagues, that concern for sleep deprivation and physician fatigue was considered.[31] However, residents' fatigue was still not seriously evaluated until 1984 when the death of a prominent newspaper columnist's daughter in New York was brought to the media forefront. Libby Zion died within 8 hours of her admission to New York Hospital, where she was cared for by first-year and second-year residents. A deadly combination of psychiatric medications was administered.[32] In 1986, a grand jury investigation ruled that her death was due to prolonged work duties and resident fatigue.[33] The Zion family's persistence led to work-hour limitations instituted by the Accreditation Council on Graduate Medical Education (ACGME) that have revolutionized modern medical education. The recommendation was for an 80-hour limit on weekly resident hours and a maximum of 24 consecutive hours on duty.[34]

In July 2003, the ACGME set national requirements, which restrict resident workweeks to a maximum of 80 hours per week, averaged over 4 weeks. Furthermore, the longest consecutive period of work cannot exceed 30 hours. Residents must have 1 day off out of 7, a minimum 10 hours off between daily work activities, and may not schedule in-house call more than 1 in every 3 nights.[35] Despite these new regulations, the Institute of Medicine concluded that 30 consecutive hours of work leads to excessive fatigue, and adjustments must be made.[36] The Joint Commission on Accreditation of Healthcare Organizations published an article in 2007[37] that also concluded that residents who work traditional schedules with recurrent 24-hour shifts (**Table 2**):

- Make 36% more serious medical errors than those whose scheduled work is limited to 16 consecutive hours[38]
- Make 5 times as many serious diagnostic errors[7]

- Have twice as many on-the-job attentional failures at night[39]
- Double their risk of a motor vehicle crash when driving home after 24 hours of work.[40] Kowalenko and colleagues[41] concluded that before residency training began, 4.1% of emergency medicine residents reported being involved in a motor vehicle collision caused by falling asleep. During their residencies, 19.3% of residents reported an accident under the same conditions
- Suffer 61% more needle stick and other sharp injuries after their 20th consecutive hour of work[42]
- Experience a 1.5 to 2 standard deviation deterioration in performance relative to baseline rested performance on both clinical and nonclinical tasks[43]
- Report making 30% more fatigue-related medical errors that led to a patient's death[44]
- Suffer decrements in performance commensurate with those induced by a blood alcohol level of 0.05% to 0.10%[45]

Table 2
Correlation between cognitive performance with sleep deprivation and ethanol intoxication

Sleep Deprivation (h)	Functional Serum Ethanol Level (%)
17–19	0.05
19–21	0.08
24	0.10

Data from Clark S. Sleep deprivation: implications for obstetric practice in the United States. Am J Obstet Gynecol 2009;201:137; with permission.

In part due to this research demonstrating risks of prolonged work hours (>24 hours), in July 2011 ACGME revised its recommendations to include that first-year residents must not work more than 16 hours. Residency programs must encourage residents to use alertness-management strategies.[46] Despite these proactive measures taken by ACGME, stricter monitoring of adherence to the rules must occur. In a Web-based survey, 84% of first-year residents reported at least 1 work-hour violation (**Table 3**).[47]

ATTENDING PHYSICIAN FATIGUE

When it comes to sleep deprivation, the adage "do as I say, not as I do" certainly applies to attending physicians. Despite creation of strict work restrictions for resident physicians, when they finish training and enter private or academic practice, there are no maximum work-hour guidelines. Typically, physicians in practice determine their own workload and lifestyle, which oftentimes leads to sleepless call nights. There has been a common belief that physicians are not significantly affected by sleep deprivation, and some reports in the medical literature have supported this misconception.[48] These studies had major flaws, including a lack of comparative controls. To presume that physicians are somehow superhuman and can function without sleep is arrogant and unsupported by quality data. Many well-designed studies of physicians who are sleep deprived demonstrate numerous effects[7]:

- Impaired language and math skills
- Poorer quality intubations
- Increased error rates in performance of laparoscopy
- Increased error rates in intensive care units
- Increased motor vehicle accidents

Table 3
Resident work hours

Category	2003 ACGME Limits	2008 IOM Recommendation	2010 ACGME Proposal
Supervision	Programs ensure supervision by qualified faculty	Supervision standards are set by a residency review committee; in-house supervision is provided for first-year residents	Residents and attendings inform patients of their roles, whereas program directors and faculty assign progressive responsibilities. Residents must have 3 levels of supervision, with a physician available to provide direct supervision for first-year residents
Workload	Assignments recognize that residents and faculty are both responsible for patient safety and welfare	Residents have adequate time for patient care and reflection. Complexity of illness and resident competency is considered in setting appropriate caseloads	Workload is based on patient safety, severity and complexity of patient cases, available support, and resident training and education
Maximum shift length	30 h (with 24 h to admit patients and 6 h for transition and educational activities)	16 h; extended duty of 30 h (with 5 h sleep after 16 continuous hours) only every third night	16 h for first-year residents; 24 h for other residents with another 4 h for transition and education. Residents must be informed of alertness strategies, and a nap is strongly suggested after 16 h of continuous duty
Minimum time off between scheduled shifts	10 h	10 h after day shift; 12 h after night shift; 14 h after extended duty period and no return before 6 AM the next day	10 h (with minimum of 8 h duty-free between shifts or 14 h duty-free after 24 h of in-hospital duty)
Mandatory off-duty time	24 h off per week averaged over 4 wk	24 h off per week, no averaging; 1 work-free weekend per month	24 h per week averaged over 4 wk; no home call on free days
Moonlighting	Internal moonlighting is considered part of the 80-h weekly limit	Internal and external moonlighting are included in the 80-h weekly limit; approval is required by program director	Internal and external moonlighting are included in the 80-h weekly limit; no moonlighting allowed for first-year residents

The Accreditation Council for Graduate Medical Education in June 2010 released proposed revisions of resident work-hour restrictions. Here is a comparison with the 2003 ACGME standards and 2008 Institute of Medicine (IOM) recommendations.

From Nasca TJ, Day SH, Amis ES Jr, et al. The new recommendations on duty hours from the ACGME Task Force. N Engl J Med 2010;363(2):e3. Available at: http://www.ncbi.nlm.nih.gov/pubmed/20573917/; with permission.

- Significant increase in family and marital stress
- Less empathy for patients
- Poorer communication to patients and family members

Obstetrics and gynecology is a field of medicine that leads to a high incidence of sleep deprivation and fatigue. The unpredictability of labor and complications thereof lend to erratic work hours and impaired sleep. In a questionnaire sent to OB/GYNs in Houston, 62 of the 100 respondents (62%) reported working greater than 80 hours per week. This value is a definite increase in hours when compared with their training.[49] In another survey of 180 physicians from primary care and surgical specialties combined, 13% of practitioners indicated they worked greater than the 80-hour work limit established for resident physicians.[50] In the limited surveys, the significant percentage of OB/GYNs who work greater than 80 hours when compared with all providers is not surprising. If residency work restrictions continue without a similar adaptation on transition to private or academic practice, the problem of sleep deprivation among physicians will continue to escalate. A physician entering a typical practice will not have had any experience during residency in working the hours now expected of him or her, thus placing patient safety at risk.

Specific to obstetrics and gynecology, the unpredictability of labor with multiple call nights spent working extended hours undoubtedly leads to abnormal sleep patterns. Over time, sleep deprivation in OB/GYN leads to job dissatisfaction and physician burnout. A study cited that the most common reason for early retirement among physicians is the desire to avoid on-call duty because of sleepless nights.[51] To support this, the Joint Commission on Accreditation of Health Organizations has concluded that "the weight of evidence strongly suggests that extended-duration work shifts significantly increase fatigue and impair performance and safety. From the standpoint of both providers and patients, the hours routinely worked by health care providers in the United States are unsafe. To reduce the unacceptably high rate of preventable fatigue-related medical errors and injuries among health care workers, the United States must establish and enforce safe work-hour limits."[37] With the rapid changes in the American health care system, physicians must take the responsibility of creating acceptable work-hour regulations before the government mandates them, as "physician work hour restrictions are likely to become more intrusive and less effective than self-imposed regulation formulated by the medical community itself."[1]

Per the National Highway Traffic Safety Administration, there are certain guidelines that may apply to physicians and could decrease the incidence of sleep deprivation with subsequent adverse patient outcomes[52]:

- Structure work to take advantage of circadian influences.
- Recognize that there is a strong urge to sleep between 3 AM and 5 AM. Avoid work that is unnecessary at this time.
- Sleep when sleepy.
- Always have backup in case of impairment due to fatigue.
- Go to sleep immediately after working a night shift to maximize sleep length.
- Recognize behaviors indicative of sleep deprivation, such as irritability.
- Apply good sleep habits. Sleep in a room amenable to quality sleep (adequate ventilation, quiet, dark, comfortable temperature).
- Use naps strategically. Do not nap more than 45 minutes to avoid deep sleep, from which it is much more difficult to awaken.

Hospitals must be proactive in supporting a safety culture. The medical staff should be educated about the effects of fatigue on patient safety. Employees should be given the opportunity to voice their concerns about fatigue.[53] A fatigue management plan that includes strategies to combat fatigue should be implemented. Some strategies may include engaging in conversations with others and performing some type of physical action throughout the work shift. Lastly, during orientation as well as on a regular basis, hospital administration should educate staff about proper sleep hygiene, including getting enough sleep, taking naps, engaging in a relaxing presleep routine (yoga, breathing exercises, reading), and avoiding food or alcohol before sleep.[54]

COMBATING SLEEP DEPRIVATION WITH A HOSPITALIST PROGRAM

The American Congress of Obstetricians and Gynecologists (ACOG) has recently taken an active role in addressing sleep deprivation and the future of the specialty. Committee Opinion #519 entitled Fatigue and Patient Safety (March 2012) provides suggestions to ensure that patient care is not compromised because of sleep deprivation among OB/GYNs. Some of the recommendations include the following[55]:

- Call schedules that provide a balance between the need for continuity of care and rest should be created.
- Alertness-management strategies should be reviewed at department meetings.
- A backup system should be available if a physician recognizes a worrisome level of fatigue.
- Consider rescheduling a surgery if the physician has been awake most of the previous night.
- Consider only working a half day or not working at all after a night on call.

Hospitalist medicine has become popular on general medicine floors so that primary care providers can focus on outpatient care and not have to manage inpatients simultaneously. Obstetricians have begun to take notice of this movement, and OB/GYN hospitalist programs are rapidly developing throughout the United States. Enacting a hospitalist system may make the aforementioned ACOG recommendations unnecessary, as OB/GYNs would be able to sleep every evening and not spend all hours of the night managing their laboring patients. OB/GYN hospitalists would perform deliveries during the evening hours, thus allowing the physicians they cover to be refreshed each morning as they prepare for office hours or the operating room. The hospitalists have no duties after their shift is done, which provides them ample rest time as well.

The term laborist was first introduced by Dr Louis Weinstein in 2003.[56] Owing to residency work-hour restrictions and the movement toward physicians choosing lifestyle over prolonged work hours, the laborist movement is quickly gaining popularity throughout the country.

Weinger and Ancoli-Israel[57] simply state that "physicians must recognize that it is neither unprofessional nor weak to admit sleepiness or fatigue when on the job and make efforts to mitigate the potential consequences to patient care." It should no longer be an embarrassment or a sign of weakness for physicians to admit that they are fatigued. In what other profession is it acceptable to boast of working prolonged consecutive hours? The badge of courage that was handed to these super physicians must now be thought of as a marker for unsafe patient care.

In 2011, the Society of OB/GYN Hospitalists (SOGH) was formed. Its mission statement is "the Society of OB/GYN Hospitalists is dedicated to enhancing the safety and quality of OBGYN Hospital Medicine by promoting excellence through education, coordination of hospital teams and collaboration with health care delivery systems". SOGH is also committed to the physician's well-being through the support and development of the OB/GYN hospitalist model.[58] Each year, attendance at the annual conference has increased, and this is a testament to the increasing acceptance of laborist programs.

Hospitalist programs are typically structured around 3 tenets: enhancing patient safety, reducing malpractice risk, and improving physician quality of life.[59] Enhancing patient safety includes both the patient and her baby. Babies born at night are 12% more likely to die.[60] Another study concluded that babies born between 2100 and 0700 are 2 times more likely to die in the first week of life.[61] Physician fatigue was referenced as a contributing factor for these increases in mortality.

A common argument against hospitalist programs is that patient satisfaction will decline because patients may object to receiving care from unfamiliar doctors. Although a legitimate concern, in the current private practice model, it is common to receive prenatal care from the same provider throughout the entire pregnancy and then be delivered by a different physician in the practice whom the patient has never met. Experience from Henrico Doctors' Hospital in Virginia, which was one of the first hospitalist programs in the country, has shown that patients quickly recognized that their safety was optimized. These women have embraced the hospitalist program with a high level of satisfaction. As we move forward in this rapidly changing health care environment, laborist programs will benefit the physicians, hospitals, and most importantly, our patients and their newborns. We must first take care of ourselves before we can ably take care of our patients. It is time for OB/GYNs to recognize that our field cannot survive with the current culture of long work hours and sleep deprivation. Furthermore, physicians from generation X and Y cite lifestyle as the single most important factor when choosing a career.[62] Continuing our current model of obstetric practice will drive our brightest medical students away from a rewarding career as an OB/GYN. Having laborists will allow physicians to have a better balance between work and family, which will ultimately lead to improved job satisfaction and better patient care.

SUMMARY

As discussed in this article, sleep deprivation is a pervasive problem affecting individuals in all occupations. Inadequate quantity or quality of sleep in pregnant women has serious medical implications that may adversely affect pregnancy outcomes. When caring for our patients, we must question their sleep habits and provide guidance in improving their sleep.

When counseling our patients regarding sleep patterns, we must also look introspectively and scrutinize our own symptoms of sleep deprivation. By providing care when fatigued, we are putting our patients, their babies, and ourselves at risk. Residency programs have strict work-hour restrictions, and it is time for attending physicians to unite and recognize the need to set guidelines for ourselves as well.

Strong consideration should be given to enacting a hospitalist program in obstetric units. This will undoubtedly lead to improved outcomes for our patients and improved quality of life for those of us caring for them. The hospitalist movement in obstetrics is still in its infancy. However, it is gaining ground throughout the country and has been widely accepted thus far.

It is hoped that obstetricians will further embrace a practice model involving laborists to improve patient safety and reduce medical errors. Quality of life for obstetricians will markedly improve, which will allow obstetrics and gynecology to continue to flourish.

Sleep that knits up the ravelled sleave of care
The death of each day's life, sore labour's bath
Balm of hurt minds, great nature's second course,
Chief nourisher in life's feast.

—William Shakespeare, Macbeth

REFERENCES

1. Eddy R. Sleep deprivation among physicians. B C Med J 2005;47(4):176–80.
2. Cirelli C. Definition and consequences of sleep deprivation. Available at: www. uptodate.com/contens/definition-and-consequences-of-sleep-deprivation. Accessed July 17, 2014.
3. Siegel JM. Sleep viewed as a state of adaptive inactivity. Nat Rev Neurosci 2009; 10:747.
4. Ohayon MM, Carskadon MA, Guilleminault C, et al. Meta-analysis of quantitative sleep parameters from childhood to old age in healthy individuals: developing normative sleep values across the human lifespan. Sleep 2004;27:1255.
5. Kirsch D. Stages and architecture of normal sleep. Available at: www.uptodate. com/contents/stages-and-architecture-of-normal-sleep. Accessed June 25, 2014.
6. Tononi G, Cirelli C. Sleep and the price of plasticity: from synaptic and cellular homeostasis to memory consolidation and integration. Neuron 2014;81:12.
7. Patrick GT, Gilbert JA. On the effects of loss of sleep. Psychol Rev 1896;3:469–83.
8. American Academy of Sleep Medicine 2008. Available at: www.aasmnet.org. Accessed December 25, 2015.
9. Young T, Skatrud J, Peppard P. Risk factors for obstructive sleep apnea in adults. JAMA 2004;291:2013–6.
10. Institute of Medicine (US) Committee on Sleep Medicine and Research, Colten HR, Altevogt BM, editors. Sleep disorders and sleep deprivation: an unmet public health problem. Extent and health consequences of chronic sleep loss and sleep disorders, vol. 3. Washington, DC: National Academies Press (US); 2006. Available at: http://www.ncbi.nlm.nih.gov/books/NBK19961/.
11. Reid K, Dawson D. Comparing performance on a simulated 12 hour shift rotation in young and older subjects. Occup Environ Med 2001;58:58–62.
12. Coulehan J, Williams PC. Vanquishing virtue: the impact of medical education. Acad Med 2001;76:598–605.
13. Knutson KL, Van Cauter E, Rathouz PJ, et al. Trends in the prevalence of short sleepers in the USA: 1975-2006. Sleep 2010;33:37.
14. Leger D. The cost of sleep-related accidents: a report for the National Commission on Sleep Disorders Research. Sleep 1994;17:84.
15. Clark S. Sleep deprivation: implications for obstetric practice in the United States. Am J Obstet Gynecol 2009;201:136.e1–4.
16. Federal Railroad Administration. The railroad fatigue risk management program at the federal railroad administration: past, present and future. Washington, DC: FRA; 2006.
17. US Code of Federal Regulations Web site. Available at: www.gpoaccess.gov/cfr/index/htm. Accessed December 25, 2015.
18. Cirelli C. Definition and consequences of sleep deprivation. In: Eichler A, editor. UpToDate. Waltham (MA): UpToDate; 2014.
19. National Sleep Foundation. 2014 Sleep in America Poll: Sleep in the Modern Family. Washington, DC: The Foundation; 2014. Available at: http://www.sleepfoundation.org/sleep-polls-data/sleep-in-america-poll/2014-sleep-in-the-modern-family.

20. Figueiro M, Bierman A, Plitnick B, et al. Preliminary evidence that both blue and red light can induce alertness at night. BMC Neurosci 2009;10(1):105.
21. Chang A, Aeschbach D, Duffy JF, et al. Evening use of light-emitting eReaders negatively affects sleep, circadian timing, and next-morning alertness. PNAS 2015;112(4):1232–7.
22. Foundation NS. Sleep in America poll. 2007. Available at: http://www.sleepfoundation.org/article/sleep-america-polls/2007-women-and-sleep. Accessed December 25, 2015.
23. Hutchison BL, Stone PR, McCowan LM, et al. A postal survey of maternal sleep in later pregnancy. BMC Pregnancy Childbirth 2012;12:144.
24. Brunner DP, Munch M, Biedermann K, et al. Changes in sleep and sleep electroencephalogram during pregnancy. Sleep 1994;17(7):576–82.
25. Bianchi MT, editor. Sleep deprivation and disease: effects on the body, brain and behavior. New York: ©Springer Science+Business Media; 2014. http://dx.doi.org/10.1007/978-1-4614-9087-6_9.
26. Klebanoff MA, Shiono PH, Rhoads GG. Outcomes of pregnancy in a national sample of resident physicians. N Engl J Med 1990;323(15):1040–5.
27. Louis J, Auckley D, Miladinovic B, et al. Perinatal outcomes associated with obstructive sleep apnea in obese pregnant women. Obstet Gynecol 2012; 120(5):1085–92.
28. Facco FL, Grobman WA, Kramer J, et al. Self-reported short sleep duration and frequent snoring in pregnancy: impact on glucose metabolism. Am J Obstet Gynecol 2010;203(2):142.e1–5.
29. Lee KA, Gay CL. Sleep in late pregnancy predicts length of labor and type of delivery. Am J Obstet Gynecol 2004;191(6):2041–6.
30. Prins JR, Gomez-Lopez N, Roberton SA. Interleukin-6 in pregnancy and gestational disorders. J Reprod Immunol 2012;95(1–2):1–14.
31. Friedman RC, Bigger JT, Kornfeld DS. The intern and sleep loss. N Engl J Med 1971;285(4):201–3.
32. Brody, JE. A mix of medicines that can be lethal. New York Times. Available at: http://www.nytimes.com/2007/02/27/health/27brody.html?n+Top/News?Health?Diseases,%20Conditions,%20and%20Health%20Topis/Antidepressants. Accessed February 27, 2007.
33. Lermer BH. A case that shook medicine: how one man's rage over his daughter's death sped reform of doctor training. The Washington Post. Available at: http://www.washingtonpost.com/wp-dyn/content/article/2006/11/24/AR2006112400985. Accessed November 28, 2006.
34. Asch DA, Parker RM. The Libby Zion case: one step forward or two steps backward? N Engl J Med 1988;318(12):771–5.
35. Accreditation Council for Graduate Medical Education. Common program requirements. 2004. Available at: www.acgme.org/acwebsite/dutyhours/dh_dutyhourscommonpr.pdf. Accessed December 25, 2015.
36. Institute of Medicine. Resident duty hours: enhancing sleep, supervision, and safety. Washington, DC: The National Academies Press; 2009.
37. Lockley SW, Barger LK, Ayas RT, et al, Harvard Work Hours, Health and Safety Group. Effects of health care provider work hours and sleep deprivation on safety and performance. Jt Comm J Qual Patient Saf 2007;33(suppl 11):7–18.
38. Landrigan CP, Rothschild JM, Cronin JW, et al. Effect of reducing interns' work hours on serious medical errors in intensive care units. N Engl J Med 2004; 351:1838–48.

39. Lockley SW, Cronin JW, Evans EE, et al. Effect of reducing interns' weekly work hours on sleep and attentional failures. N Engl J Med 2004;251:1829–37.
40. Barger LK, Cade BE, Ayas NT, et al. Extended work shifts and the risk of motor vehicle crashes among interns. N Engl J Med 2005;352:125–34.
41. Kowalenko T, Kowlenko J, Gryzbowski M. Emergency resident related auto accidents – is sleep deprivation a risk factor? Acad Emerg Med 2000;7:1171.
42. Ayas NT, Barger LK, Cade BE, et al. Extended work duration and the risk of self-reported percutaneous injuries in interns. JAMA 2006;296:1055–62.
43. Philibert I. Sleep loss and performance in residents and nonphysicians: a meta-analytic examination. Sleep 2005;28:1392–402.
44. Barger LK, Ayas NT, Cade BE, et al. Impact of extended-duration shifts on medical errors, adverse events, and attentional failures. PLoS Med 2006;3:e487.
45. Arnedt JT, Owens J, Crouch M, et al. Neurobehavioral performance of residents after heavy night call vs. after alcohol ingestion. JAMA 2005;294:1025–33.
46. Nasca TJ, Day SH, Amis ES Jr. The new recommendations on duty hours from the ACGME Task Force. N Engl J Med 2010;363:e3.
47. Landrigan CP, Barger LK, Cade BE, et al. Interns' compliance with Accreditation Council for Graduate Medical Education work-hour limits. JAMA 2006;296:1063–70.
48. Gaba DM, Howard SK. Patient safety: fatigue among clinicians and the safety of patients. N Engl J Med 2002;347:1249–55.
49. Promecene PA, Schneider KM, Monga M. Work hours for practicing obstetrician-gynecologists: the reality of life after residency. Am J Obstet Gynecol 2003;189(3):631–3.
50. Chen I, Vorona R, Chiu R, et al. A survey of subjective sleepiness and consequences in attending physicians. Behav Sleep Med 2008;6:1–15.
51. Katz JD. Issues of concern for the aging anesthesiologist. Anesth Analg 2001;92:1487–92.
52. National Transportation Safety Board. Factors that affect fatigue in heavy truck accidents. NTSB Safety Study NTSB/SS-95/01. Washington, DC: NTSB; 1995.
53. The Joint Commission Sentinel Event Alert. Issue 48, December 14, 2011.
54. Rosekind MR, Gander PH, Connell LJ, et al. Fatigue countermeasures: alertness management in flight operations. National Aeronautics and Space Administrations, Southern California Safety Institute Proceedings. Long Beach (CA), 1994.
55. Fatigue and patient safety. Committee Opinion No. 519. American College of Obstetricians and Gynecologists. Obstet Gynecol 2012;1229:683–5.
56. Weinstein L. The laborist: a new focus of practice for the obstetrician. Am J Obstet Gynecol 2003;188(2):310–2.
57. Weinger M, Ancoli-Israel S. Sleep deprivation and clinical performance. JAMA 2002;287(8):955–7.
58. Available at: www.societyofobgynhospitalists.com. Accessed December 25, 2015.
59. Dunnavant S. Changing times, changing practices. The doctor's advocate. First quarter 2013.
60. Gould JB, Qin C, Chavez G. Time of birth and the risk of neonatal death. Obstet Gynecol 2005;106(2):352–8.
61. Borland S. Babies born at night three times more at risk for death. MailOnline. Available at: www.dailymail.co.uk/news/article-1295149/Babies -born-night-times-higher-risk-death.html. Accessed July 16, 2010.
62. Weinstein L, Garite T. On call for obstetrics – time for a change. Am J Obstet Gynecol 2007;196(1):3.

Obstetrics Hospitalists
Risk Management Implications

Larry Veltman, MD, CPHRM, FACOG

KEYWORDS

- OB hospitalist • In-house obstetrician • Laborist • Risk management
- Perinatal safety net • Obstetric emergencies

KEY POINTS

- In-house obstetricians provide a safety net for management of obstetric (OB) emergencies that may require expertise and rapid intervention in order to adequately respond to these situations.
- There are emerging data that the presence of OB hospitalists on a perinatal unit improves maternal and newborn outcomes.
- There is a broad spectrum of activities that allows OB hospitalists from any given model to participate in risk management activities at multiple levels in the organization.

RISK MANAGEMENT, CLAIMS, GETTING TO HAVARTI

Risk management has evolved as an independent discipline and profession that is based on the classic concepts of loss prevention and loss reduction.[1] Hospitals generally have an individual designated as a risk manager. This individual may have an independent position or may have other combined duties within the patient safety or quality components of the organization. A significant part of hospital risk management is the management of medical malpractice claims. According the American Society of Healthcare Risk Management, obstetrics (OB) continues to be a leading source of severity of medical malpractice claims.[2] Results of the 2012 Professional Liability Survey conducted by The American College of Obstetricians and Gynecologists (ACOG) showed that neurologically impaired infant claims were the most common claim against obstetricians (28.8% of 2564 claims), stillbirth or neonatal death was the second most common claim (14.4% of 2564 claims), and delays or failure to diagnose were allegations in 11.1% of these claims. The respondents were asked in the survey to identify other factors that applied to OB claims. These factors included

Disclosures: There are no commercial or financial conflicts of interest or funding sources to report.
205 Southeast Spokane Street, Suite 320, Portland, OR 97202, USA
E-mail address: l.veltman@comcast.net

Obstet Gynecol Clin N Am 42 (2015) 507–517
http://dx.doi.org/10.1016/j.ogc.2015.05.008
0889-8545/15/$ – see front matter © 2015 Elsevier Inc. All rights reserved.

obgyn.theclinics.com

electronic fetal monitoring (20.9%), shoulder dystocia/brachial plexus injury (15.1%), and interactions with OB-gynecology (GYN) residents (11.4%).[3]

Getting to Havarti is a metaphor that this author has advanced for improving safety in the perinatal unit.[4] The Swiss cheese model of James Reason[5] is an important concept describing how accidents occur in complex organizations such as labor and delivery units. Reason's[5] model suggests that when failures in existing defenses and safeguards coincide, the trajectory of a potential accident can penetrate all of these accident protections to cause an injury. The idea of making the holes in the Swiss cheese smaller (ie, getting to Havarti; a Danish cheese with very small holes) is a metaphor for targeting certain areas of a perinatal unit to tighten defenses and safeguards so the chance of penetration by an accident's trajectory is reduced and most often deflected. The idea of placing an obstetrician in house, 24 hours a day, 7 days a week, is one recommendation that theoretically should tighten a perinatal unit's defenses (therefore reducing the size of the holes) and subsequently reduces the chance for patient injury. This safety net offers one of the best risk management loss prevention strategies available to a perinatal unit, particularly to labor and delivery.

Common Obstetric Practices That Can Weaken Defenses

What makes the holes in the Swiss cheese larger?

- The obstetrician may need to be in 3 or 4 places at once. Because of the demands of an OB-GYN practice, an obstetrician can be scheduled in the operating room, the office, and have patients in labor at 1 hospital, and sometimes 2 hospitals, at the same time.
- High-volume practice. Booking a large number of patients that might be delivering at more than 1 hospital puts stress on the practitioner's ability to see all of these patients in the office as well as attend all of the deliveries.
- Poor sign-out practices. Multiple providers caring for 1 patient can sometimes result in confusion about changes in the patient's condition or who is in charge of the patient's care at any given time.
- Inadequate protocols for consultation, referral, or transfer. This situation can result in confusion and, at times, variation in the timing and the nature of consultation between midwives, family physicians, obstetricians, and perinatologists.
- Acquiescing to patient requests that are may be unsafe. There can be the temptation, at times, to yield to pressure from patients; for example, to perform an elective induction earlier than 39 weeks or to allow a trial of vaginal birth after caesarean when there may be inadequate immediately available personnel or operating room space available during a trial of labor after cesarean within the hospital.
- Off-site monitoring of high-risk situations. The demands of an office practice, the operating room, or the need for sleep can sometimes take the physician away from the patient's bedside during a critical situation.
- Operation of hierarchy and the lack of teamwork when it comes to safety issues. OB care has come to be recognized as a team effort and there are occasions when not listening to safety concerns of nurses or house staff can result in failed recognition of a potential problem.
- Backup may be inadequate. Because of the nature of the practice group or the call sharing agreements (or lack of such) within the community, obstetricians may find that they are without backup to care for patients when they are otherwise occupied.

- Failure to recognize the ability of human factors to impair vigilance. Sometimes physicians find themselves on call for long periods of time. There is ample evidence about the adverse effects of fatigue on the ability to make decisions in health care.[6,7]

The Hospitalist Movement

In 1996, Wachter and Goldman[8] described a model of care in which hospital-based physicians provided patients' inpatient care in lieu of the patient's primary physician. They termed these physicians hospitalists. The hospitalist movement has taken hold and, by 1999, 65% of internists had hospitalists in their community and 28% reported using them for inpatient care.[9] In 2003, Louis Weinstein,[10] in an article entitled, "The Laborist: A New Focus of Practice for the Obstetrician," advocated the adoption of the hospitalist model to OB care. In a 2010 study of 28,545 members of the ACOG contacted in a national survey, 7044 clinicians responded, which yielded a response rate of 25%. Of the respondents, 1020 clinicians (15% of respondents, 3.6% of the sample) described themselves as OB/GYN hospitalists or laborists.[11] According to the Web site (www.obgynhopsitalist.com), there are at least 241 hospitals in the country that use a laborist or OB hospitalist model of care.[12]

How Does an Obstetrics Hospitalist Program Function as a Safety Net for a Perinatal Unit?

Can the patient's physician not always be available and in-house during the patient's labor? Because there are many aspects of OB practice that may require the physician to be away from labor and delivery during some portion of a given patient's labor, the answer is often No. As aptly stated by Clark and colleagues[13]:

> Obstetrics today is a team process, requiring the coordinated, integrated involvement of physicians, midwives, nurses, technicians, laboratory support personnel, and the mother. ...Obstetrics in the United States is, (however)...unique in that the traditional captain of the team is often not present during important parts of the labor process.

In addition, there is the human factor of fatigue that, at times, interfaces with the OB workload. This workload, including night call, could require a particular obstetrician to be available for multiple successive nights to manage the labors of multiple patients. With regard to fatigue and its association with a possible deleterious effect on patient safety, a recent ACOG Committee Opinion recommends that, "all practitioners ... address fatigue, and efforts should be made to adjust workloads, work hours, and time commitments to avoid fatigue when caring for patients."[14]

Can the establishment of in-house coverage with an OB hospitalist model improve patient safety and reduce claims of malpractice? Clark and colleagues,[15] in 2008, addressed this issue with the following:

> A review of almost 200 closed malpractice claims demonstrated that 40% of adverse outcomes related to intrapartum fetal hypoxia, and their associated malpractice claims, may have been avoided had such (in-house) coverage been available.

Physicians, nurses, and risk managers have all recognized that in-house OB hospitalists can serve as an important safety net for patient care in a variety of ways, including:

- Decreasing the chance for precipitous deliveries while the patient's own provider is in transit.

- Acting as a liaison between nurses and physicians when there is concern about a potential unsafe practice.
- Rescue of a newborn from an abruption or ruptured uterus by performing an emergency cesarean delivery.
- Offering to give second opinions to both nurses and physicians.
- Stepping in as an assistant for surgery and assisting with other OB emergencies, such as shoulder dystocia or postpartum hemorrhage.
- Providing the immediate availability of an OB surgeon for trials of labor after cesarean deliveries.
- Providing backup for midlevel providers.
- Participating in nursing education.
- Assuming leadership roles in drill and simulation design and debriefings.
- Providing emergency call coverage for patients without physicians who present to the emergency department (ED) or to the labor unit.

An example of such an intervention is a case of a primiparous patient laboring at 41 weeks' gestation with reassuring fetal heart tracing showing normal baseline and variability, frequent accelerations, and normal uterine activity pattern. As the labor became more active at approximately 6 to 7 cm slightly after midnight the fetal heart tracing showed a prolonged deceleration, which proceeded to a sustained bradycardia with loss of variability. This pattern persisted over the next 10 minutes during transfer of the patient to the operating suite while the attending obstetrician was being called in from home. The OB hospitalist then initiated the cesarean section and delivered a fetus with Apgar scores of 7 at 1 minute and 9 at 5 minutes as the attending was arriving. The arterial cord pH was 7.13, affirming the appropriateness and importance of early intervention and management (Duncan Neilson, MD, Medical Director, Women's Health Services, Legacy Health System, Portland, OR, personal communication, 2008).

Is There Objective Evidence That Obstetrics Hospitalists Improve Outcomes and Reduce the Chance for Adverse Outcomes?

Given that adverse events in OB are rare, it takes a considerable number of deliveries over time to show that there is benefit in outcomes from any particular intervention. However, there are some studies of maternal and neonatal outcomes that have examined the role of OB hospitalists as a primary intervention as well as several additional studies that have incorporated OB hospitalists or in-house call as part of an overall perinatal safety program.

In 2013, Srinivas and colleagues[16] studied 626,772 patients delivered in 24 hospitals. Implementation of laborists resulted in fewer labor inductions, reduced maternal prolonged length of stay, and decreased term neonatal intensive care unit admissions. In addition, there was a significant reduction in preterm delivery.

A theoretic model based on a hospital with 1000 deliveries per month found that the addition of a 24-hour laborist model of coverage would have resulted in improved fetal outcomes. In a population of 100,000 women, 24-hour OB coverage resulted in a reduction of 47.1 neonatal deaths per year, 38.4 stillbirths per year, and 24.9 fewer cases of neurologic developmental delay.[17]

Barber and colleagues[18] showed that a change to a night float (providing in-house physician coverage at night) was associated with a decreased use of induction of labor, an increased likelihood of using oxytocin, and a decreased likelihood of performing manual extraction of the placenta or episiotomy. There were also fewer third-degree and fourth-degree lacerations and fewer neonates born with an umbilical artery pH of less than 7.10.

Gosman and colleagues[19] showed that establishment of a rapid response team (of which an in-house maternal-fetal medicine [MFM] specialist or hospitalist was a component) resulted in an increased use of this team for various OB emergencies.

In addition, 2 studies of comprehensive patient safety initiatives from Yale–New Haven Hospital and New York Weill Cornell Medical Center showed a decrease in overall adverse outcomes. The presence of in-house obstetricians was a component of each of these initiatives.[20,21]

Despite these promising studies and a wealth of anecdotal experience, there is a continued need to establish objective evidence that there is a risk management benefit to implementing an OB hospitalist program. Attempts to separate the OB hospitalist program from other perinatal safety activities, examination of a large number of deliveries, and multiple institution trials should occur to firmly establish the value of the OB hospitalist movement.[22]

THE OBSTETRICS HOSPITALIST MOVEMENT AND MODELS OF CARE

An important consideration that is directly related to patient safety involves the benefits of the OB hospitalist model to the lifestyle stresses and human factors that affect the practice of OB. The practice of OB frequently involves extensive multitasking, working when fatigued, time pressures, sacrificing valued family time, and concern that any error may precipitate litigation. This stress may lead to what has been termed burnout. It has been shown that in cases of physician burnout there is an association with an increased chance for errors.[23] Desirable aspects of the OB hospitalist model, as opposed to a more traditional OB/GYN practice model, include regularly scheduled shifts, more control in the work hours (and therefore less fatigue), and guaranteed time off.[10]

Several models have been successful in creating in-house coverage. Every model has some of the same challenges and issues in establishing this type of coverage. These issues include the number of FTEs (Full time equivalents), professional fees or salaries, billing practices, credentialing, professional liability coverage, and the scope of practice of OB hospitalists. At one end of the spectrum of coverage is to contract with an organization that provides an entire team of OB hospitalists to cover a given perinatal unit. At the other end of the spectrum, the existing community medical staff agrees to provide in-house coverage of the unit on a rotating basis. This coverage by the community obstetricians can be compensated or voluntary. There are multiple models that exist along this continuum as alternatives. For example, a hospital may recruit individual OB hospitalists from the community (either locally or nationally) or a hospital could contract with an individual group of obstetricians in the community who agree to provide hospitalist coverage for the unit. There are several Web sites and resources that can be accessed to determine the best model for a given perinatal unit's volume and makeup. (for example, www.societyofobhospitalists.com; www.obgynhospitalist.com; www.obhg.com).

OVERCOMING CHALLENGES/THE ROLE OF THE RISK MANAGER

There are multiple challenges associated with establishing a successful OB hospitalist program regardless of the model that is chosen. Risk managers can help overcome these challenges by using patient safety as a central theme. Whether the challenge is the business case for safety, patient and provider satisfaction, or the establishment of appropriate policies and procedures, risk managers should take the opportunity to bring the safety aspects of such a program into focus for the entire perinatal and administrative team.

Cost

It is clear that any organization considering the addition of OB hospitalists must address the costs of such a program. Specifically, when it comes to assessing cost and examining the business case for safety, risk managers should work with senior management to gain buy-in regarding the economic impact of adding an OB hospitalist model. With respect to recouping the costs of such a program, a 2008 study conducted by the Advisory Board estimated that, at a volume of approximately 1000 deliveries per year, a perinatal unit, with active billing procedures, could come close to breaking even for the necessary costs of the additional FTEs.[24] It is sometimes difficult to prove prospectively that savings will occur with respect to the OB rescues, decreased liability, and fewer missed deliveries that the OB hospitalist model promises. However, risk managers, with anecdotes and available data, should play an important role in framing the business case in terms of added safety.

Patient Satisfaction

Depending on the OB hospitalist model, patient satisfaction may or may not become an issue. It is common and understandable that patients usually want their physicians or midwives to be involved with their delivery. Because care by group practices often divides call between physicians in the practice, it is common, even without hospitalists, to have physicians or midwives other than the patient's primary caregiver involved with care in labor and delivery. Framing the introduction of the OB hospitalists in terms of patient safety is the best strategy when introducing the OB hospitalist team to the community and individual patients. Many models of OB hospitalist coverage do not include the hospitalist doing deliveries for private patients except in emergencies, but do allow for hospitalist's compassionate support and interventions during labor if the patient's primary caregiver is out of the hospital.

Provider Satisfaction

Challenges to the implementation of an OB hospitalist program may occur from providers, nursing staff, and administration. Education regarding rescues, reminding how in-house physicians can prevent accidents; continued participation in analysis of adverse events and near misses; and ongoing awareness and distribution of literature with regard to OB hospitalists serve to advance the cause of this safety net.

Perceived threats that physicians or midwives will be excluded from their own patients' care are common with the initiation of OB hospitalist programs, but soon dissipate as the safety elements of the program become real and the true role of the hospitalist becomes common knowledge. Clinicians who have practiced OB for many years have all missed deliveries, felt the anxiety of having to be in 2 or more places at once, and wished for an immediate assistant in an unexpected emergency. As these situations are addressed and rescues occur from having a skilled physician who is always in the hospital, the perceived threats to autonomy are likely to disappear.

Establishment of Policies and Procedures Surrounding the Obstetrics Hospitalist Model

The leadership of the perinatal department (or division of OB) should form a multidisciplinary team (to include hospital risk managers) that remains focused on policies, procedures, and operational models to improve patient safety. The OB hospitalist model needs to be integrated into the operational structure of the unit. Clarity about the scope of practice, the limitations of interventions, and communications throughout all levels of the unit need to be established with new policies and procedures.

A key element for instituting an obstetric... hospitalist program within a facility is the establishment of clear communication methods between...hospitalists and primary health care providers. Handoff of patients, updates on progress, and follow-up, are all important areas to address because communication gaps are a potential source of patient injury.[25]

There are multiple policies that need clear definition. These include issues of safety (eg, a patient is admitted to the hospital for induction, and the OB hospitalist is asked to intervene by rupturing membranes but does not think the induction is timely or indicated; what communications between providers need to take place to resolve this conflict?), issues of billing practices (eg, the hospitalist stands by for a potential delivery for a physician in transit but the physician arrives just in time to deliver his or her own patient; is that a billable event?), and issues that define the scope of practice of the OB hospitalist (eg, what if a physician wants the OB hospitalist to care for a patient in the hospital but the OB hospitalist thinks that the patient should be transferred to a higher level of care?). Clearly not every contingency can be addressed in a given policy but a departmental committee that includes all stakeholders should be established to resolve such conflicts if and when they arise.

In considering the role of OB hospitalists as an important step toward improving patient safety in OB, the following endorsement from the 2010 Committee Opinion of the ACOG should be kept in mind:

... the American College of Obstetricians and Gynecologists supports the continued development of the obstetric-gynecologic hospitalist model as one potential approach to achieving increased professional and patient satisfaction while maintaining safe and effective care across delivery settings.[25]

The Defined Duties of a Hospitalist From a Sample Contract

- Maintain high visibility in the department, maintain awareness of clinical activity on the OB unit, and have no other clinical or administrative responsibilities during the clinical shift.
- Collaborate with the charge nurse in ensuring safe and efficient daily operations, proactively discuss concerns for patient safety, and function as defined in the chain of command policy for the unit.
- Adhere to and support established clinical protocols, identify potentially better practice, and work to implement clinical change and quality initiatives.
- Foster collaborative teamwork among all health care providers in the unit, while behaving in an exemplary professional manner.
- Arrange postdischarge follow-up for unassigned patients or unassigned patients seen in triage by the hospitalist service.
- Remain aware of labor and delivery patient census and activity throughout the assigned coverage period, including:
  - Handover at change of shift with hospitalist going off duty and charge nurse
  - Review of patient census with the charge nurse at least twice during shift
  - Periodic assessment of triage patient activity
  - Periodic assessment of electronic patient census and fetal tracings on all monitored patients as necessary
- Admit, manage, deliver, and provide postpartum care for unassigned patients during labor and delivery.

- In consultation with MFM, admit, manage, deliver, and provide antepartum and postpartum care for preterm patients during labor and delivery and/or those patients with significant comorbidities.
- Provide medical coverage for triage and ensure that patients are not discharged from triage without predischarge medical review by the attending physician or the hospitalist.
- Communicate triage issues to the attending by phone as necessary and fax evaluations to the attending office in a timely manner.
- Assist with unscheduled cesarean sections when available.

ED responsibilities for GYN patients:

- Respond to ED for phone consultation or clinical evaluation for unassigned patients not requiring admission.
- Provide clinical evaluation, initiation of admission history, physical examination, and orders for unassigned gynecologic patients coming to the ED requiring admission (using the backup laborist for OB duties if necessary).
- Perform emergency gynecologic surgery procedures as OB workload permits (using the backup laborist for OB duties if necessary).

Responsibilities for departmental quality and safety:

- Adhere to current practice guidelines, standing orders, and improvement initiatives, including those related to infection control, accreditation, and regulatory requirements.
- Advocate for evidence-based safety and consistency in practice.
- Work collaboratively with departmental leadership to identify opportunities for quality, safety, or operational improvement through standardization, guideline development, or work process improvement.
- Support the nursing staff as appropriate in review and interpretation of fetal heart tracing and labor progress. This role is intended as an educational support to help the nurses improve appropriate use of the nomenclature, interpretation skill, and clarity in reporting patient status to attending physicians. Maintain a collegial relationship with staff relative to offering support for clinical decision making.
- Be familiar with the unusual occurrence report (UOR) process and purpose. Support completion of UORs as mechanisms to identify quality improvement opportunities.
- Lead real-time critical incident debriefs on cases in which they are involved.
- Participate in safety rounds and so-called huddles with charge nurses, anesthesia clinicians, and staff.
- Be available for OB emergencies, whether assisting the attending or providing direct management in the absence of the attending physician.
- Understand the role in chain of command and execute responsibility per chain of command policy.
- Be familiar with essential hospital and OB policies, guidelines, and protocols including but not limited to:
  - Universal protocol
  - Medication reconciliation
  - Smoking cessation
  - Drug testing
  - Human immunodeficiency virus testing
  - Hand washing

- o Infection control
- o Electronic fetal monitoring nomenclature
- o Oxytocin administration protocol
- o Massive fluid transfusion protocol (when developed)
- o Magnesium administration protocol: tocolysis and pregnancy-induced hypertension

Additional Responsibilities and Expectations:

- Promote patients' satisfaction with their experience of care, support a culture of safety, and meet behavioral expectations to create an environment conducive to mutual respect and learning between physicians and staff. Recognize the significance of being the face of the OB unit for patients, attending physicians, and staff. These behaviors are characterized by:
  - o Collaboration
  - o Responsiveness
  - o Timeliness
  - o Customer service orientation
  - o Consensus building
  - o Team work
  - o Use of SBAR (Situation, background, assessment, recommendation) structured communication
  - o Pleasant, calm disposition in an environment in which uncertainty is present and the ability to multitask is required
  - o Electronic fetal monitoring nomenclature and competency training
  - o Team training
  - o Critical incident debriefing training
  - o Simulation training
  - o Communication/SBAR
  - o Managing difficult people/critical conversations
  - o Review of policies and procedures
  - o Competency training for use of electronic medical record

EARLY RESOLUTION, APOLOGY, AND DISCLOSURE

In the last several years, strategies advocating early discussion and resolution, apology, and disclosure associated with unexpected outcomes have become important risk management precepts. Thirty-seven states have passes so-called apology laws that, to some degree, prohibit expressions of empathy (and in some states, fault) to be admissible in trials[26]; Massachusetts and Oregon have initiated early discussion and resolution legislation,[27,28] and multiple health care systems and professional liability carriers have provided data that the approach to identification of adverse outcomes, early discussions with patients, apology, and disclosure offers significant benefit to the patient, the providers, and the financial picture of these organizations.[29] OB hospitalists, through their inpatient presence and involvement with patient care, especially in emergencies, may have objective observations and insight into the issues surrounding an adverse outcome. Through appropriate training, leadership skills, and engagement of other members of the medical staff (who may be reluctant to become involved in these risk management approaches to an adverse outcome), OB hospitalists are in a unique position to participate in any of these patient interaction approaches as a result of establishing a strong relationship with the hospital's risk management department.[30]

SUMMARY

Most outcomes in OB are normal. However, emergencies do occur and any adverse outcome with respect to a mother or newborn can be devastating to the family, the caregivers, and the institution. Emergency management requires a culture of preparedness and availability of resources. An in-house obstetrician, be it an obstetrician from the community or an independent OB hospitalist, fits well with a major risk management precept, that of loss prevention, in the ability to provide a safety net that provides expertise and eliminates delays in care.

REFERENCES

1. Orlikoff J, Vanagunas A. Malpractice prevention and liability control for hospitals. Chicago (IL): American Society of Health Systems; 1988.
2. American Society of Healthcare Risk Management. Pearls for obstetrics. Chicago (IL): American Society for Healthcare Risk Management of the American Hospital Association; 2012.
3. ACOG. Professional liability survey, 2012. Available at: http://www.acog.org/About-ACOG/ACOG-Departments/Professional-Liability/2012-Survey-Results. Accessed November 1, 2014.
4. Veltman L. Getting to Havarti: moving toward patient safety in obstetrics. Obstet Gynecol 2007;110:1146–50.
5. James R. Managing the risks of organizational accidents. Hampshire (England): Ashgate Publishing; 1997.
6. Available at: www.rapplaw.com/library/fatigue-and-medical-m.cfm. Accessed June 4, 2007.
7. Feyer AM. Fatigue: time to recognise and deal with an old problem: it's time to stop treating lack of sleep as a badge of honour [Editorial]. Br Med J 2001; 322(7290):808–9.
8. Wachter RM, Goldman L. The emerging role of "hospitalists" in the American health care system. N Engl J Med 1996;335:514–7.
9. Auerbach AD, Nelson EA, Lindenauer PK, et al. Physician attitudes toward and prevalence of the hospitalist model of care: results of a national survey. Am J Med 2000;109:648–53.
10. Weinstein L. The laborist: a new focus of practice for the obstetrician. Am J Obstet Gynecol 2003;188:310.
11. Funk C, Anderson BL, Schulkin J, et al. Survey of obstetric and gynecologic hospitalists and laborists. Am J Obstet Gynecol 2010;203:177.e1–4.
12. Available at: www.obgynhospitalist.com. Accessed December 9, 2014.
13. Clark SL, Belfort MA, Byrum SL, et al. Improved outcomes, fewer cesarean deliveries, and reduced litigation: results of a new paradigm in patient safety. Am J Obstet Gynecol 2008;199:105.e1–7.
14. Fatigue and Patient Safety. ACOG committee opinion no. 398. American College of Obstetricians and Gynecologists. Obstet Gynecol 2008;111:471.
15. Clark SL, Belfort MA, Dildy GA. Reducing obstetric litigation through alterations in practice patterns experience with 189 closed claims. Am J Obstet Gynecol 2006; 195:S118.
16. Srinivas S, Macheras M, Small D, et al. Does the laborist model improve obstetric outcomes? American Journal of Obstetrics and Gynecology, Supplement, S1–S438. 34th Annual Meeting of the Society for Maternal-Fetal Medicine: The Pregnancy Meeting, Sandiego, CA, February 16, 2013. 210:S48.

17. Allen A. The cost effectiveness of 24 hr in-house obstetric coverage. American Journal of Obstetrics and Gynecology, Supplement, S1–S438. 34th Annual Meeting of the Society for Maternal-Fetal Medicine: The Pregnancy Meeting, Sandiego, CA, February 13, 2013. 210:S48.
18. Barber EL, Eisenberg DL, Grobman WA. Type of attending obstetrician call schedule and changes in labor management and outcome. Obstet Gynecol 2011;118:1371–6.
19. Gosman GG, Baldisseri MR, Stein KL, et al. Introduction of an obstetric-specific medical emergency team for obstetric crises: implementation and experience. Am J Obstet Gynecol 2008;198:367.e1–7.
20. Pettker CM, Thung SF, Lipkind HS, et al. A comprehensive obstetric patient safety program reduces liability claims and payments. Am J Obstet Gynecol 2014;211: 319–25.
21. Grunebaum A, Chervenak F, Skupski D. Effect of a comprehensive obstetric patient safety program on compensation payments and sentinel events. Am J Obstet Gynecol 2011;204(2):97–105.
22. Srinivas K, Lorch SA. The laborist model of obstetric care: we need more evidence. Am J Obstet Gynecol 2012;207(1):30–5.
23. Shanafelt TD, Balch CM, Bechamps G, et al. Burnout and medical errors among American surgeons. Ann Surg 2010;251(6):995–1000.
24. Advisory Board. Laborist program breakeven analysis. Washington, DC: The Advisory Board; 2008.
25. The Obstetric-Gynecologic Hospitalist. Committee opinion no. 459. American College of Obstetricians and Gynecologists. Obstet Gynecol 2010;116:237–9.
26. Saitta N, Hodge S. Efficacy of a physician's words of empathy: an overview of state apology laws. J Am Osteopath Assoc 2012;112(5):302–6.
27. Available at: http://oregonpatientsafety.org/discussion-resolution/. Accessed December 31, 2014.
28. Available at: http://www.massmed.org/News-and-Publications/MMS-News-Releases/Landmark-Agreement-Between-Physicians-and-Attorneys-Provides-for-Medical-Liability-Reforms-in-Massachusetts/. Accessed December 31, 2014.
29. Kachalia A, Kaufman SR, Boothman R, et al. Liability claims and costs before and after implementation of a medical error disclosure program. Ann Intern Med 2010;153:213–21.
30. Hendrich A, McCoy CK, Gale J, et al. Ascension Health's demonstration of full disclosure protocol for unexpected events during labor and delivery shows promise. Health Aff (Millwood) 2014;33(1):39–45.

Organizing an Effective Obstetric/Gynecologic Hospitalist Program

Christopher Swain, MD[a],*, Mark Simon, MD, MMM[a],
Brian Monks, MD[b]

KEYWORDS

- Obstetric-gynecologic hospitalist • Hospitalist programs • Obstetric emergencies
- Patient safety • Clinical support

KEY POINTS

- An obstetric/gynecologic (OB/GYN) hospitalist may provide a broader level of service, encompassing both obstetric and gynecologic patients within the entire hospital and the emergency department.
- Effective communication is a necessary component of any successful OB/GYN hospitalist program.
- The OB/GYN hospitalist program start-up process should be smooth and straightforward so as to gain credibility during a very stressful time of initial uncertainty.
- The obstetric emergency department is a foundational aspect of an OB/GYN hospitalist program.
- If implemented properly, managed well from an operational/fiduciary perspective, and adequately used, an OB/GYN hospitalist program should be a very cost-effective safety initiative.

INTRODUCTION

The obstetric/gynecologic (OB/GYN) hospitalist care model is a rapidly growing phenomenon within the specialty of obstetrics and gynecology. It is mirroring the popularity of the original hospitalist model introduced in a 1996 *New England Journal of Medicine* article by Wachter and Goldman[1] within the specialty of internal medicine. Unlike a laborist, who typically cares only for obstetric patients in the labor and delivery (L&D) unit, an OB/GYN hospitalist may provide a broader level of service,

Disclosures: The authors are employees of Ob Hospitalist Group, Inc.
[a] Ob Hospitalist Group, Inc, 10 Centimeters Drive, Mauldin, SC 29662, USA; [b] Ob Hospitalist Group, Ob Hospitalist, North Austin Medical Center, 12221 North Mo-Pac Expressway, Austin, TX 78758, USA
* Corresponding author.
E-mail address: cswain@obhg.com

Obstet Gynecol Clin N Am 42 (2015) 519–532
http://dx.doi.org/10.1016/j.ogc.2015.05.009
0889-8545/15/$ – see front matter © 2015 Elsevier Inc. All rights reserved.

obgyn.theclinics.com

encompassing both obstetric and gynecologic patients within the entire hospital and the emergency department (ED).

The current environment for OB/GYNs and for hospitals providing OB/GYN services is a challenging one, because of the following:

- Decreasing reimbursements
- Heavy call burden/high patient volumes
- Decreasing levels of job satisfaction/retention for L&D nurses and staff obstetricians
- Decreased quality of life for OB/GYNs
- Oppressive medico-legal environment
- Increasing demands on physician time and hospital resources

The OB/GYN hospitalist model has been proposed as a solution to many of these challenges. As noted in the American College of Obstetricians and Gynecologists Committee Opinion No. 459, the OB/GYN hospitalist model has the potential to provide benefits to practicing obstetrician-gynecologists, to hospitals, nurses, patients, and their families. "The American College of Obstetricians and Gynecologists supports the continued development of the OB/GYN hospitalist model as one potential approach to achieving increased professional and patient satisfaction while maintaining safe and effective care across delivery settings."[2] Although it is obvious that the immediate availability of emergency obstetric services translates into improved patient safety in the face of catastrophic emergencies, there are many opportunities to investigate a vast array of other benefits that may be provided by an OB/GYN hospitalist program.

The operative word in the preceding paragraph is "potential." In reality, many hospitals across this country have considered implementing OB/GYN hospitalist programs but have chosen not to do so because they could not clearly determine how effective these programs would actually be for their women's health service line. Others have attempted to start programs but these ultimately failed for a variety of reasons. Quite frankly, the implementation of OB/GYN programs is no simple matter. Many components must be considered and managed during the start-up process as well as the operational phase of programs to ensure success.

Essentially, successful OB/GYN hospitalist programs must meet the following 3 very important goals:

- Reducing liability exposure by improving patient safety and clinical outcomes
- Generating enough revenue to avoid being a financial liability
- Providing clinical support to the staff or private OB/GYNs without being competitive

The more effective and successful programs are those that have achieved the greatest amount of confluence between these stated goals (**Fig. 1**).

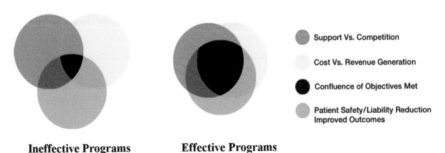

Ineffective Programs   **Effective Programs**

Fig. 1. Effective versus ineffective OB/GYN hospitalist programs. (*Courtesy of* © 2015 Ob Hospitalist Group.)

How can one OB/GYN hospitalist program flourish while another struggles? Most likely, the program that is successful has considered and managed the components of its program better. A thorough understanding of these various components, along with their proper utilizations, will likely be the best and most reliable predictor of a successful program.

This article addresses the various components of an OB/GYN hospitalist program in an effort to illustrate how proper development and management can result in the formation of a more effective program.

CLINICAL EXCELLENCE

First and foremost, the OB/GYN hospitalist is an emergency responder who will react to any obstetric or gynecologic emergency within the hospital. Additionally, there are other core functions that are commonplace in most OB/GYN hospitalist programs:

- Obstetrics triage unit management
- Evaluation and management of unassigned obstetric patients
- Management of unassigned gynecologic emergencies
- Surgical assistant for cesarean deliveries

To perform these functions, the OB/GYN hospitalists should be experienced, board-certified physicians with impeccable reputations among their peers and favorable malpractice histories. There is no universal standard with regard to how many years of clinical experience is required before a provider is felt to be suitable for this role; however, a general consensus is that board certification, together with at least 5 years of full-time clinical experience, is sufficient. The OB/GYN hospitalist must be experienced enough to competently and calmly manage a wide variety of patient-care scenarios and obstetric emergencies, while also thoroughly understanding the doctor-patient relationship, operational aspects of hospitals, and the complexities of managing a private practice. The successful hospitalist must be service-minded, as a genuine spirit of service to patients, clinicians, and hospital is critical to the success of an OB/GYN hospitalist program.

An OB/GYN hospitalist team is more effective if composed of physicians who do not have practice affiliations within the community. This staffing practice creates a dedicated, neutral team that is not viewed as competition by community physicians, thus resulting in greater utilization of the program. The OB/GYN hospitalist team should be selected by decision-making hospital representatives after personal interviews and thorough consideration of their credentials. They also should be required to successfully complete various training modules, such as the following:

- Advanced fetal monitoring interpretation
- Operative vaginal delivery techniques
- A recognized program to improve teamwork and communication, such as Team STEPPS (teamwork system developed by the Department of Defense)
- Management of obstetric emergencies, such as shoulder dystocia management and evaluation/management of postpartum hemorrhage
- Advanced cardiac life support/neonatal resuscitation program certification

Effective communication is a necessary component of any successful OB/GYN hospitalist program. Patient handoffs occur regularly between OB/GYN hospitalists and primary physicians; appropriate management of transitions of care is essential to patient safety, and is conducive to a healthy partnership between hospitalists and primary physicians. The Joint Commission estimates that 80% of serious medical errors involve miscommunication between caregivers when responsibility for patients is transferred or handed-off.[3] An OB/GYN hospitalist program, to be successful, should have a well-defined protocol outlining physician-to-physician communication processes surrounding patient handoffs, and a reliable mechanism for obtaining prenatal records from within the offices of the staff obstetricians for enhanced continuity of care purposes.

TEAM LEADER PHYSICIAN OR MEDICAL DIRECTOR

The interactions among the OB/GYN hospitalists, staff obstetricians, L&D nurses, patients, and hospital administrators must be considered as core operational components of any program. To enhance these interactions, a team leader physician or medical director should be chosen who will be responsible for team management duties, such as the following:

- Coordinating the schedule for the team of OB/GYN hospitalists
- Serving as a liaison between OB/GYN hospitalist team members, hospital representatives, and a management company (if applicable)
- Actively participating in various departmental meetings of the hospital

The team leader/medical director will enable one team member to better represent his or her fellow OB/GYN hospitalists and promptly address any problems or concerns that might arise with regard to an individual's performance. **Fig. 2** is an example of the reporting structure for OB Hospitalist Group, a privately owned national OB/GYN

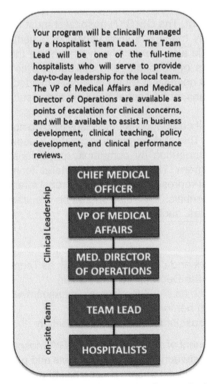
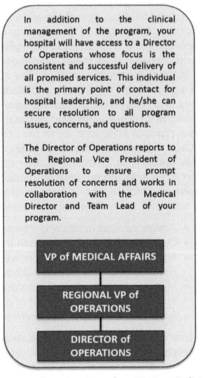

Fig. 2. Example of team leader/medical director reporting structure for OB Hospitalist Group. MED, medical; VP, vice president. (*Courtesy of* © 2015 Ob Hospitalist Group.)

hospitalist program. As demonstrated here, the team leader/medical director is supported and supervised by a hierarchy of other physician leaders, as well as operational support personnel within the company. An OB/GYN hospitalist program independently operating and housed within a hospital will likely also have a team leader/medical director who reports to the hospital's vice president of medical affairs. Simultaneously, all hospitalists also are held accountable to the individual hospital's medical staff through the medical executive committee and the peer-review structure.

WELL ORGANIZED START-UP PROCESS

The OB/GYN hospitalist program start-up process should be detailed and comprehensive. It also should be well understood by all involved parties to ensure that the program's initiation is timely and uneventful. The importance of this process cannot be overemphasized. A smooth and straightforward start-up is essential because it enables the program to gain credibility during a very stressful time of initial uncertainty. A successful program implementation makes the transition to an OB/GYN hospitalist program much more reassuring and satisfying for all parties involved. Features of this process should include most, if not all, of the items shown in **Box 1** and **Fig. 3**.

PATIENT EDUCATION/PREPAREDNESS

To facilitate an effective patient-care team, it is important that patients be educated to anticipate the potential involvement of the OB/GYN hospitalist in their hospital care even before a program begins. The OB/GYN hospitalists may be introduced as practice "associates" who are continuously at the hospital to enhance patient safety. Some practitioners introduce the hospitalist concept by assuring the patient that "I, or one of my associates, will be at the hospital 24 hours a day, 7 days a week, to assist you." The American College of Obstetricians and Gynecologists recognizes the OB/GYN hospitalist model as a potential solution to achieving increased patient satisfaction.[2] Hospitalist experience to date has shown that patients appear to be very willing to trade familiarity (of their primary doctor) for availability/competency (of the hospitalist) when it comes to hospital care.[4]

CUSTOMIZATION/PRIORITIZATION OF PROGRAM DESIGN BASED ON THE FACILITY'S NEEDS

From the administrative perspective, a hospital will typically be most concerned about improving the following items:

- Patient safety
- Clinical support for its providers and resident physicians
- Morale of its clinical staff (including nurses)
- Productivity of its physicians

Although hospitals are unique in many ways, they often share common goals regarding care ideals and the success of health care service lines. Many hospitals share recognizable deficiencies in women's health service line. A fairly comprehensive list of these deficiencies is noted in **Box 2**.

Successful programs are not simply "cookie-cutter" models or designs. Instead, they should be thoughtfully designed, facilitating a unique partnership between the hospital, the medical staff, and the OB/GYN hospitalist team. By providing a variety of customized services, an OB/GYN hospitalist program can remedy many deficiencies within hospitals while providing a host of potential benefits (**Box 3**).

Box 1
Guidelines for an obstetrician/gynecologist (OB/GYN) hospitalist program start-up process

1. Program Start-Up Management

   A. Review, refine, and communicate program "start-up plans"

   B. Provide overall implementation guidance and direction throughout the onboarding phase for all stakeholders involved in launching the new program

   C. Manage, track, and provide status of the implementation activities to promote timely and complete transition to the new program

   D. Conduct regular project team meetings (conference calls) to keep all participants aligned and accountable for completing assigned tasks

2. Program Set-up

   A. Customize program procedures, forms, and policies to comply with the hospital's requirements/expectations

   B. Define, develop, and implement an obstetric emergency department (OB ED) with the hospital

   C. Provide sample scoring guides, charge sheets, and other relevant OB ED documentation

3. Physician (Hospitalist) Recruiting

   A. Perform all hospitalist recruitment activities, including advertising, candidate identification, and initial screenings

   B. Complete candidate interviews, background reviews, and qualification verifications (eg, certificates, licenses)

   C. Schedule and participate in the hospitalist interviews with the hospital team

   D. Collaborate with hospitals to ensure each prospective hospitalist completes the required application and privileging documentation

4. Stakeholder Communications and Preparations

   A. Participate in initial hospital departmental meetings to address program-specific operational and clinical questions

   B. Conduct or participate in program-specific discussions with local/staff physicians to address patient and clinical questions

Courtesy of © 2015 Ob Hospitalist Group.

OBSTETRIC EMERGENCY DEPARTMENT

The obstetric ED (OB ED) is a foundational aspect of an OB/GYN hospitalist program that deserves special attention. This key component of a viable OB/GYN hospitalist program involves the transformation of the L&D triage unit into an OB ED. The L&D triage unit is typically the only acute patient-care area within hospitals in which patients are not routinely examined and managed by physicians. Many hospitals simply have nurses evaluate the OB patients in the triage unit of L&D with assessments given to the on-call obstetrician via the phone. Verbal telephone orders are then given by the physician. Patients often are managed and discharged in this manner with the physicians never physically evaluating them. This model of care is commonly referred to as "nurse triage" or "telephone triage," and it consistently has been associated with more liability exposure for hospitals and OB/GYNs, as well as low levels of patient and nurse satisfaction.

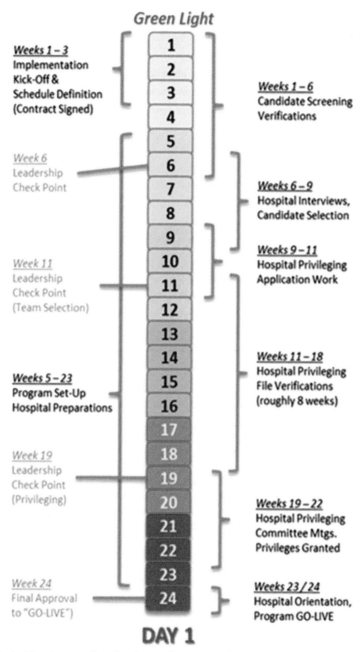

Green Light

Weeks 1–3
Implementation
Kick-Off &
Schedule Definition
(Contract Signed)

Weeks 1–6
Candidate Screening
Verifications

Week 6
Leadership
Check Point

Weeks 6–9
Hospital Interviews,
Candidate Selection

Week 11
Leadership
Check Point
(Team Selection)

Weeks 9–11
Hospital Privileging
Application Work

Weeks 5–23
Program Set-Up
Hospital Preparations

Weeks 11–18
Hospital Privileging
File Verifications
(roughly 8 weeks)

Week 19
Leadership
Check Point
(Privileging)

Weeks 19–22
Hospital Privileging
Committee Mtgs.
Privileges Granted

Week 24
Final Approval
to "GO-LIVE")

Weeks 23/24
Hospital Orientation,
Program GO-LIVE

DAY 1

Fig. 3. Typical implementation timeframe. (*Courtesy of* © 2015 Ob Hospitalist Group.)

An OB ED remedies this disparity in care by requiring that all unscheduled patients presenting to L&D be evaluated by a team of a nurse and either a physician or advanced care nurse before being discharged. This change increases patient and nurse satisfaction/retention[5] while also creating a new source of revenue for the

---

Box 2
Common deficiencies in women's health service line

- Lack of immediately available obstetric emergency care
- Insufficient management of obstetric triage patients
- Need improved process to manage unassigned obstetric patients
- Need improved process to manage unassigned gynecologic patients
- No emergency preparedness drills
- Lack of surgical assistants for cesarean deliveries
- Insufficient midwife support
- Insufficient proctoring of family practice residents
- Family practitioners need additional support
- Unable to perform vaginal birth after cesarean
- Inability to perform timely OB/GYN consults
- Need to develop a high-risk service
- Difficulties recruiting and retaining new obstetricians
- Obstetric nursing dissatisfaction and turnover
- Diminished productivity of staff OB/GYN physicians

Courtesy of © 2015 Ob Hospitalist Group.

---

hospital, because it can now appropriately capture ED facility charges rather than outpatient or triage unit charges for these unscheduled problem visits.

An OB ED requires a physician or advanced care nurse to be physically available to the OB ED at all times. This requirement is typically met by the OB/GYN hospitalists but, on the rare occasions when these providers might be involved in the care of other patients off the L&D unit, it is advisable for staff physicians to provide backup support or coverage for the hospitalists via a rotational call schedule. The staff OBs, in return for their backup coverage, would have all unassigned patients needing outpatient care referred to them. The consistent 24/7 presence of a clinician in L&D enables emergencies to be handled much more expeditiously and reduces overall hospital malpractice exposure.[6] It also helps to remedy alleged delays of care. "Delay in treatment of fetal distress" is a very common allegation in lawsuits and a significant issue that threatens patient safety. A 2000 to 2009 retrospective study done by The Doctors Company showed that this was the major allegation in at least one-half of all neonatal brain damage and death cases.[7] Malpractice liability reduction, together with the new revenue generated from an OB ED, are the most important factors in enabling hospitals to offset the costs of an OB/GYN hospitalist program.

CLINICAL SUPPORT/EDUCATION

The presence of an OB/GYN hospitalist on the labor unit creates ongoing opportunities for education and support. This ready availability allows for the following:

- Improved emergency preparedness by enhancing the timely response of a clinician
- Availability to participate in mock drills and educational seminars

---

Box 3
Customized services and potential benefits of an OB/GYN hospitalist program

Proposed Customizable Services	Potential Program Results and Benefits
• 24/7 On-site OB/GYN hospitalist coverage	• Risk management
	○ Malpractice liability reductions
• OBED program management and leadership	○ Malpractice reserve reductions
• Business development support	• Business development
• Patient safety program initiatives and collaborations	○ Physician retention and recruitment
	○ Local clinic partnerships
• Hospitalist malpractice coverage	○ Midwifery group support (if applicable)
• Main emergency department consult availability	○ On-site clinics
	○ Transport services
• On-site clinics and community clink partnerships	• Operational expense reduction
• Residency program management and proctoring	○ Reduction in unnecessary admissions
	○ Improved nursing efficiencies
• Midwifery support	○ Improvement of nurse retention
• Management of transport patients	• Service revenue
• Reporting and analytics services	○ Labor and delivery facility revenue
• Facility billing reconciliation	○ Neonatal intensive care unit utilization and expansion
• Hospitalist recruitment and placement services	○ Peripheral revenue
• Call coverage for local physicians	
• Drills, training, and simulations	

Courtesy of © 2015 Ob Hospitalist Group.

- Availability to assist with the training of nurses, medical students, and residents
- Rapid access of non-OB/GYN obstetric providers to an OB/GYN specialist

An OB/GYN hospitalist also can perform many other vitally important functions for his or her assigned hospital. In particular, the OB/GYN hospitalist can help improve the productivity and efficiency of staff obstetricians and perinatologists by providing them with a variety of support services. Having an OB/GYN hospitalist program often allows hospitals to eliminate a daily physician-on-call expense, as the OB/GYN hospitalists will assume primary responsibility for unassigned patients. Also, many hospitals realize savings related to the proctoring of residents and medical students, using the OB/GYN hospitalists to provide this supervision.

MATERNAL FETAL MEDICINE SUPPORT

The office workload for many perinatologists makes it very difficult for these providers to manage an inpatient population. Increasingly, a number of these perinatal subspecialists are focusing primarily on outpatient duties. An OB/GYN hospitalist team could comanage these high-risk patients in partnership with the maternal fetal medicine (MFM) team. This symbiotic relationship or partnership enables

- MFMs to focus on consultative services rather than direct patient care issues
- More high-risk patients to be cared for or managed at a given hospital instead of being referred elsewhere
- Hospitals to easily accept maternal-fetal or high-risk obstetric patient referrals and transports

Most MFMs are not readily available to assist with emergency preparedness drills in L&D. The OB/GYN hospitalists, however, can facilitate regular performance of clinical drills to help the clinical staff (nurses and physicians) prepare for OB emergencies and meet the objective of the Joint Commission that advocates using mock OB emergency training drills as a risk-reduction strategy.[8]

STAFF OBSTETRIC SUPPORT

The private or staff OBs can be more productive in their offices by reducing unnecessary trips to the hospital to manage routine patient care needs. The OB/GYN hospitalists can

- Review questionable fetal heart rate tracings
- Place intrauterine pressure catheters/fetal scalp electrodes
- Perform amniotomies
- Monitor patients after epidural placement/order epidurals
- Supervise patients attempting vaginal birth after cesarean during their labors
- Evaluate postpartum bleeding
- Place/remove and manage intrauterine tamponade balloons
- Supervise oxytocin augmentation
- Stand in for unattended deliveries

In a typical scenario, the private physician, whether at home or in the office, continues to be the "captain of the ship" regarding the management of the laboring patient, with the OB/GYN hospitalist playing only a supporting role. This model of in-house coverage also satisfies the requirement for immediate physician availability for trial-of-labor patients and allows hospitals to offer this option to patients instead of simply recommending repeat cesarean delivery to their patients or having some patients go to a different, competing hospital for a trial of labor. This form of coverage also could help reduce a hospital's overall cesarean delivery rate.[9]

A 2002 study of medical hospitalists by Wachter and Goldman[4] reported that "the average primary care physician would realize a yearly net gain of about $40,000 by forgoing hospital care, simply by replacing wasted commute time with increased ambulatory productivity." OB/GYN hospitalists can essentially function as "silent partners," allowing the staff OBs more time to complete office duties, perform GYN surgeries, or get a few more hours of sleep. These providers also can provide some call coverage and patient rounding support for the staff OBs, which would further enhance their lifestyles and help to reduce burnout. This level of support allows private physicians to periodically sign-out their inpatient service to the OB/GYN hospitalist team, permitting the OB/GYN hospitalists to take over as the "captain of the ship," and, thereby, managing all patient care decisions. Such support activities, quite importantly, need to be noncompetitive in nature so as to facilitate physician engagement and utilization. These physician support services promote enhanced recruitment of new physicians, as well as improved retention of current providers. OB/GYN hospitalist support allows staff physicians to take care of more patients in their offices, with the hospital ultimately benefiting from an increased service volume. The provision of more extensive physician support services, however, must be dependent on the service/patient-care volume and safe availability of the OB/GYN hospitalist.

OBSTETRIC SERVICE AGREEMENTS

OB/GYN hospitalist teams frequently provide inpatient call coverage for staff physicians. In return for this type of coverage, a nominal fee is charged to the private obstetrician. This fee, although small, reminds the staff OBs that these services have inherent value and minimizes excessive or abusive use of the OB/GYN hospitalists. Such coverage arrangements can have significant billing and collection consequences if done improperly. It is recommended that this type of obstetric call support should be done under a formal contractual arrangement (an obstetric service agreement, for example).

NATIONAL QUALITY FORUM AND QUALITY METRICS MONITORING

Compliance with risk management initiatives and National Quality Forum (NQF) metrics is important to hospitals, because these initiatives can improve safety, reduce malpractice risk, and improve reimbursements from third-party payers (**Table 1**). Well-defined initiatives and thoughtful management can be the difference between a failing and a thriving program. Noncompliance with these standards can result in decreased payments or declined claims for hospitals. A fully engaged OB/GYN hospitalist program can help hospitals to achieve and measure quality metrics. The core measures of a program should be monitored and measured on an ongoing basis.

STRATIFICATION OF SUPPORT INITIATIVES

An effective OB/GYN hospitalist program is a comprehensive, stratified model of support and function that is customized to serve the unique needs of the hospital. The program must have different strategies and support mechanisms built into its infrastructure to maximize its effectiveness. These enhancements, if used properly, can be extremely valuable tools for maintaining alignment between the hospitalist providers and the hospital representatives, ensuring that all stated objectives for the program are being met satisfactorily (**Fig. 4**).

COST CONSIDERATIONS

Cost is the principal factor restricting implementation of OB/GYN hospitalist programs. Professional revenue alone will typically not be able to fully offset the expense of a program. Additional sources of new or "downstream" revenue always must be

Table 1	
National Quality Forum (NQF) metrics	
NQF 469	Elective deliveries <39 wk gestation
NQF 470	Episiotomy rate
NQF 471	NTSV with cesarean delivery
NQF 472	Antibiotic prophylaxis within 1 h for cesarean delivery
NQF 473	DVT prophylaxis for cesarean delivery
NQF 476	Initiation of antenatal steroids for gestational age 24–31 6/7 wk
NQF 477	Number of births less than 1500 g, if applicable (hospitals without a Level 3 NICU)
NQF 1746	GBS prophylaxis

Abbreviations: DVT, deep vein thrombosis; GBS, group B streptococcal; NICU, neonatal intensive care unit; NTSV, nulliparous term singleton vertex.
Courtesy of © 2015 Ob Hospitalist Group.

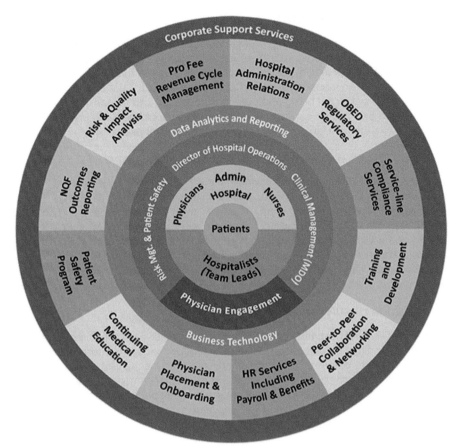

Fig. 4. An effective model of support mechanisms built into the infrastructure of the OB/GYN hospitalist program. HR, human resources. (*Courtesy of* © 2015 Ob Hospitalist Group.)

considered when evaluating the cost-effectiveness of programs of this type. Some of these key financial drivers have been previously introduced in this article, but they bear repeating because of the huge impact they have on the overall financial performance of OB/GYN hospitalist programs:

- OB ED facility revenue
- Elimination of on-call stipends paid to staff OBs for unassigned patient coverage
- Malpractice liability and reserve reductions
- Expansion of perinatal and maternal transport services
- Expansion of neonatal intensive care unit services
- Increased delivery/obstetric patient volume
- Increased elective GYN surgery volume due to enhanced productivity of staff physicians
- Call coverage/support for staff OB/GYN providers
- Reduction in unnecessary admissions
- Proctoring of residents and medical students

An OB/GYN hospitalist program has many potential mechanisms to generate the quality and revenue necessary to justify and sustain its existence (**Fig. 5**). These

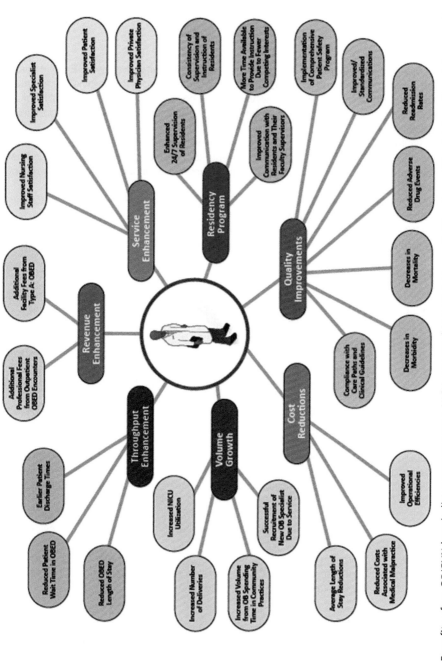

Fig. 5. Benefits of an OB/GYN hospitalist group program. NICU, neonatal intensive care unit. (*Courtesy of* The Advisory Board Company.)

mechanisms will vary greatly from hospital to hospital, and a true cost analysis must consider the impact of multiple variables.

If implemented properly, managed well from an operational/fiduciary perspective, and adequately used, an OB/GYN hospitalist program should be a cost-effective safety initiative.

SUMMARY

The thoughtful development and implementation of a comprehensive OB/GYN hospitalist program can result in a cost-effective practice model that provides increased value through a wide variety of services. The continuous on-site availability of an OB/GYN specialist affords many benefits to patients, hospitals, and practicing physicians.

A well-implemented and effective OB/GYN hospitalist program will be associated with many different service line improvements for hospitals. Such programs increase patient safety, promote risk reduction, and improve clinical outcomes, while enriching the quality of life of OBs and GYNs.

The OB/GYN hospitalist model is a trend that is likely to see increasingly wide adoption in the coming years. Careful consideration of the design and implementation of an OB/GYN hospitalist program as described in this article will set the stage for success and help to facilitate the continued growth and expansion of this model going forward.

REFERENCES

1. Wachter R, Goldman L. The emerging role of "hospitalists" in the American health care system. N Engl J Med 1996;335(7):514–7.
2. The American College of Obstetricians and Gynecologists. Committee opinion no. 459: the obstetric-gynecologic hospitalist. Obstet Gynecol 2010;116(1):237–9.
3. Zhani E. Joint Commission center for transforming healthcare tackles miscommunication among caregivers. 2010. Available at: http://www.centerfor transforminghealthcare.org/news/detail.aspx?ArticleId=294153. Accessed April 29, 2012.
4. Wachter RM, Goldman L. The hospitalist movement 5 years later. JAMA 2002;287: 487–94.
5. Wolfe S. Hospitalists: good or bad for nurses? RN 2000;63(3):31–3.
6. Clark SL, Belfort MA, Dildy GA, et al. Reducing obstetric litigation through alterations in practice patterns. Obstet Gynecol 2008;112(6):1279–83.
7. Ranum D. A study of OB claims. Seminar/PowerPoint presented to the society of OB/GYN hospitalists. Denver (CO). August 31, 2011.
8. Joint Commission on Accreditation of Healthcare Organizations: Sentinel event alert. Issue 30, July 21, 2004. Available at: http://www.jointcommission.org/assets/1/18/SEA_30.PDF.
9. Klasko SK, Cummings RV, Balducci J, et al. The impact of mandated in-hospital coverage on primary cesarean delivery rates in a large non-university teaching hospital. Am J Obstet Gynecol 1995;172:637–42.

Business and Organizational Models of Obstetric and Gynecologic Hospitalist Groups

Thomas J. Garite, MD[a,b,*], Lisa Levine, MD, MSCE[c], Rob Olson, MD[d]

KEYWORDS

- OB/GYN hospitalist programs • Patient safety • Program costs • Patient satisfaction
- Malpractice coverage

KEY POINTS

- Hospitalists have done well in patient satisfaction surveys, indicating a willingness among hospital administrators to provide subsidies for initiating obstetric and gynecologic (OB/GYN) hospitalist programs.
- Some hospitals have experienced indirect changes from OB/GYN hospitalist programs that have improved their bottom line.
- The principal hurdles or difficulties for OB/GYN hospitalist programs are funding, training, staffing, private physician acceptance, patient acceptance, and malpractice coverage.

BUSINESS AND ORGANIZATIONAL MODELS OF OBSTETRIC AND GYNECOLOGIC HOSPITALIST GROUPS

The burgeoning growth of obstetric and gynecologic (OB/GYN) hospitalists throughout the United States over the past decade has led to a number of ways to approach how groups of OB/GYN hospitalists are organized. The organizational and business models do, however, depend on what one's perception of what an OB/GYN hospitalist is. A recent survey (Levine LD, Schulkin J, Mercer B, et al, American Journal of Perinatology, in press.) illustrates just how diverse is the idea of what

[a] University of California, Irvine, Building 22 - Route 81, 101 The City Drive, Mail Code: 3200, Orange, CA 92668, USA; [b] Obstetrics MedNax/Pediatrix Medical Group, Perigen Inc, Sunrise, FL, USA; [c] Department of Obstetrics and Gynecology, Perelman School of Medicine, University of Pennsylvania, Philadelphia, PA, USA; [d] Society of OB/GYN Hospitalists, Peace Health St. Joseph Medical Center, ObGynHospitalist.com, Bellingham, WA, USA
* Corresponding author. University of California, Irvine, Building 22 - Route 81, 101 The City Drive, Mail Code: 3200, Orange, CA 92668.
E-mail address: tjgarite@uci.edu

Obstet Gynecol Clin N Am 42 (2015) 533–540
http://dx.doi.org/10.1016/j.ogc.2015.05.010
0889-8545/15/$ – see front matter © 2015 Elsevier Inc. All rights reserved.

defines an OB/GYN hospitalist. Among general OB/GYN physicians and Maternal Fetal Medicine (MFM) specialists, 68% defined an OB/GYN hospitalist or laborist as a member of a group providing 24/7 coverage on labor and delivery and not having a separate office practice, whereas 20% defined an OB/GYN hospitalist or laborist as having an office practice but covering either his or her own practice's patients in shifts on labor and delivery or covering unassigned and other physician's patients as well. Thus, the concept of an OB/GYN hospitalist or laborist is not only different in different practitioners' minds, but the organization of such different models can be very different from one program to another.

If we as a specialty are going to realize all the advantages of OB/GYN hospitalist practices, however, we must recognize that practitioners who do this as just 1 piece of their practice, within the context of a separate outpatient practice, are not really fulfilling the promise of what this new specialty can deliver in terms of patient safety, patient satisfaction, optimal communication among nurses and physicians, and the desires of obstetrician gynecologists to have a more balanced life style. Because those individuals with office practices who also do occasional dedicated labor and delivery coverage have their own business models (usually some variants of private group practice), the remainder of this article is devoted to how organizational and business models of OB/GYN hospitalists are structured for those physicians whose professional practice is devoted entirely to inpatient obstetrics with or without emergency room and/or inpatient gynecology coverage.

The business and organizational structures of OB/GYN hospitalists are not unlike those of other hospitalists, emergency room, anesthesia, and intensive care unit physicians, which have a substantially longer history. Like these other groups, there is a diversity within this new specialty of how they are structured and how they become financially solvent. The reasons for the differences in these organizational structures are multiple. First is the reason a hospital chooses to initiate an OB/GYN hospitalist group. The reasons for setting up such a new program often are multiple for any given hospital and may include the following:

- History of poor obstetric outcomes on the unit (with or without associated malpractice lawsuits) thought to be owing to physicians who are not immediately available or owing to poor nurse–physician communication aggravated by lack of availability
- The need to cover certified nurse midwife services and family practitioners who provide obstetric care
- Difficulty in providing care for obstetric emergency room or obstetric triage patients
- The need to provide in-house supervision for obstetric residents
- The need to provide services to "dropin" patients and unassigned patients as well as those who present in advanced labor or with critical needs
- The need to provide inpatient services for MFM physicians who often are busy with outpatient consultations and ultrasounds and may prefer not to take (or want to reduce) night call
- Individuals or groups of physician obstetric providers who need coverage assistance with their obstetric patients during busy office hours or on nights and weekends

A second and evolving reason for initiating an OB/GYN hospitalist program, especially among staff model programs such as Kaiser Permanente, is the desire for physician "tracking," where some physicians prefer office-only care, others gynecologic surgery, and still others labor and delivery and inpatient care. Some of this is driven by lifestyle preferences and needs, but also by a lack of sufficient gynecologic surgery cases for the members of the entire group to maintain skills and privileges.

The third set of reasons for differences in types of OB/GYN hospitalist groups relate to the cost of initiating and maintaining such a program. Depending on a number of factors, including the size of the obstetric service, payer mix, and private physicians' interest in having the hospitalists, OB/GYN hospitalists generally do not generate enough revenue to cover the cost of their salaries and malpractice premiums and benefits, especially for the first 2 to 3 years. Thus, the shortfall will have to be subsidized by the group or institution hiring them. OB/GYN hospitalists' costs can be recovered in a variety of different ways. Reimbursement for the deliveries they do can be substantial, especially if private physicians are passing off a moderate percentage of their deliveries to the hospitalists. Reimbursement will be inadequate if the OB/GYN hospitalists are covering only midwife deliveries and/or "dropin" patients. There are other sources of revenue depending on the specific hospital setting. These can include the following:

- Billing professional fees for triage/obstetric emergency room evaluations, including ultrasound and fetal monitoring evaluations (often billed separately as non-stress tests)
- Covering gynecologic emergency room patients and performing or assisting on emergency surgery on these patients
- Assisting on cesarean sections and other procedures requiring a second physician, such as twin deliveries
- Doing morning rounds for private physicians or MFMs
- Being the primary physicians who accept and care for maternal transports
- Performing procedures in labor and delivery such as external cephalic versions, amniocenteses, or amnioreductions

Regardless, many of these sources of revenue, especially in dominantly private practice obstetric units, will depend to a great extent on the willingness of private physicians to share their patients with the OB/GYN hospitalists. It takes time for the private physicians to overcome their fears of losing their patients, poor patient satisfaction, and of being ultimately relegated to ambulatory care only providers.

An OB/GYN hospitalist program will often have to be subsidized (at least in the short term) and, in many cases, indefinitely. However, hospitals that hire or subsidize OB/GYN hospitalists yield a number of benefits not seen in immediate gain in patient revenue. These include the following:

- Having a physician or physicians who can perform administrative duties and lead patient safety teams
- Improved nursing satisfaction, retention, and even hiring
- Relief from having to pay for coverage of other obstetric and administrative services
- Enhanced bedside teaching and impromptu or formal conference teaching for nurses and trainees
- Labor and delivery problem solving and administrative duties
- Ease in developing and implementing protocols, check lists, drills, and simulation
- Better supervision of house staff
- Less hassle with private physicians over having to provide emergency room coverage
- Helping triage elective admissions during busy times
- More ease in coverage of nurse midwives, family physicians, and "dropin" patients

- Lower cesarean section rates[1,2]

In addition, some hospitals have experienced indirect changes from OB/GYN hospitalist programs that have improved their bottom line with such things as increased attraction of new private physicians and patients, thereby increasing delivery volume, reducing malpractice risk and claims, increasing or improving flow of maternal transports, and decreasing nursing staff turnover. Hospitalists, in general, have done well in patient satisfaction surveys.[3] Thus, there is a willingness among many hospital administrators to provide subsidies for initiating OB/GYN hospitalist programs, at least in the short run.

The job of running a hospitalist program is complex. There are many administrative considerations that must either be in place or developed to initiate and sustain a new program. "Human resource" activities include recruiting and hiring, establishing credentials of new hires, patient billing, credentialing the new hospitalists with the hospital and insurance plans, providing benefits and malpractice insurance, payroll, staffing for vacations and illnesses, dealing with turnover, performance evaluations, and so on. The day-to-day running of the program and ensuring all the hospitalists and those who depend on the work of the hospitalists are satisfied with the services they are providing. Whichever model for organizing, compensating, and managing the new group of OB/GYN hospitalists will result in a substantial amount of administrative and financial challenges.

How are OB/GYN hospitalist practices organized? Surveys differ somewhat according to whom is surveyed and when the survey was done. According to a recent survey (Levine LD, Schulkin J, Mercer B, et al, American Journal of Perinatology, in press.) of general OB/GYNs and MFMs, OB/GYN hospitalists employment models include employment by the hospital or university in 41% to 49%, self-employment in independent groups in 12% to 17%, employment as part of a private practice (general or multispecialty group) in 12% to 18%, as physician practice management groups in 5% to 10%, as an MFM group 2% to 10%, and other in 6% to 10%.

Advantages and disadvantages vary for various types of hospitals. In university programs, which have been relatively positive about adopting OB/GYN hospitalist programs, the advantages are somewhat different. Most university programs provide in-house attending physician coverage and have residents and attendings on the units at all times. The primary motivation for adding an OB/GYN hospitalist service here is quite different. Often physicians from the subspecialty divisions, especially the reproductive endocrinology and infertility, gynecologic oncologists, and urogynecologists, do not want to have to provide coverage on labor and delivery units. There are financial advantages and improved recruitment and retention if the MFM faculty do not cover labor and delivery. MFM practices are more profitable and MFM providers are happier covering daytime ambulatory services on high-risk patients, performing ultrasounds and outpatient procedures while limiting labor and delivery coverage to consultations and primary care for selected patients. Another motivation at university hospitals is that, by allowing a group of physicians to focus on labor and delivery, there is a group of knowledgeable and skilled providers who are better care givers and teachers for this specific area. Many teaching hospitals, including university services, have private physician services as well and hospitalists who can provide services for and derive revenue from their private patients.

Hospitals with staff models of physician coverage have other motivations for developing hospitalist type services, as discussed, and these services tend, at least to date, to be hybrid services covered by a mixture of OB/GYN hospitalists as well as other OB/GYN physicians who do not limit their duties to labor and delivery. For many of these hospital-owned and run OB/GYN hospitalist programs, the malpractice insurance of the hospital may provide, or provide at less cost, the insurance for the hospitalists and thus provide an economy not provided in other models.

In many ways, independent OB/GYN hospitalist groups are like other hospital-based specialties, such as anesthesiology or emergency room physicians. They develop administrative, human resources, billing, and clerical infrastructures of their own or contract with the hospital or private companies to perform these duties. This is no small task for a group of only 4 to 6 physicians covering 1 hospital. Usually, such groups are heavily subsidized by the hospital and/or the hospital may provide the infrastructure for the financial, human resources, and administrative duties in turn for which the OB/GYN hospitalists may provide some administrative and other duties for the hospital in the form of a medical director of the OB/GYN hospitalist service. Although surveys suggest that this is a relatively common model (Levine LD, Schulkin J, Mercer B, et al, American Journal of Perinatology, in press.), it is speculated that many of these independent groups have relationships with the hospital that mitigate some of the costs and challenges of running a private practice and thus are a hybrid between a true independent private practice and a hospital-based practice, but with more autonomy than a purely hospital owned and run practice.

Four Physician Practice Management Companies provide the bulk of this type of practice model in the United States. The largest and only exclusively OB/GYN hospitalist program is the "Ob Hospitalist Group" (www.obhg.com).[4] Currently OBHG manages practices in more than 70 hospitals around the United States. MedNax (mednax. net)[5] and its division of the Pediatrix/Obstetrix Medical Group currently has 10 OB/GYN hospitalist practices, some as extensions of their MFM practices and others free standing. This company is a large physician practice management company that manages neonatal, MFM, pediatric subspecialty, and anesthesia practices and well as OB/GYN hospitalist practices. Two other groups, Delphi or Team Health (www.teamhealth.com) and Quest Care (www.questcare.com)[6,7] manage several different types of hospitalist practices, and also manage a relatively small number of OB/GYN hospitalist programs. These national professional organizations take over the burden of the administrative issues of running a physician practice from the hospital in return for a management fee. With the economies of scale provided to administrative and HR services, malpractice insurance, and other centralized functions, these groups can often provide OB/GYN hospitalists to the hospital at a lesser initial cost, with less startup risk and considerably less difficulty recruiting, staffing, and retaining OB/GYN hospitalist physicians. These companies also have the advantage of a larger pool of physicians who can provide coverage of both temporary and permanent positions. The larger companies are also are likely to have more extensive experience with billing and coding, resulting in enhanced revenue capture as well as experience in developing and running OB/GYN hospitalist programs.

The final model is the OB/GYN hospitalist who functions either exclusively or partly as an MFM extender. As well-described by D'Alton and colleagues,[8] in an article entitled "Putting the "M" back in MFM," the evolution of the subspecialty of MFM has been away from the inpatient care of maternal obstetric complications, focusing instead more on the outpatient setting with fetal diagnosis and therapy, ,genetics and consultative obstetrics. This development has been driven by 2 main forces: the greater profitability of outpatient practice and lifestyle issues allowing MFM physicians to avoid night and weekend work. Furthermore, the main reason MFM groups tend to hire new MFM physicians is often owing to the increasing burden of night and weekend call. The salary of an MFM physician, even a new fellowship graduate, is considerably higher than an OB/GYN hospitalist. Many services, including maternal transports, deliveries of premature babies, and management of "high-risk" patients who successfully avoid major complications are successfully managed by a well-trained OB/GYN hospitalist guided by protocols developed in conjunction with MFM.

Interestingly, we are not aware of a model of private groups of multispecialty hospitalists or of inpatient physicians forming groups, to take advantage of common infrastructure among types of practices that do not provide ambulatory services.

We have discussed the advantages of each of these types of organizational structures, but what are the disadvantages of each? To date, only physicians who are dedicated inpatient OB/GYN hospitalists with no other practice or office practice have been shown to benefit care, principally and so far by lowering cesarean section rates and increasing the number of patients electing to have a trial of labor after previous cesarean section.[1] We limit the discussion to the latter model of OB/GYN hospitalists. The principal hurdles or difficulties for OB/GYN hospitalist programs are funding, training, staffing, private physician acceptance, patient acceptance, and malpractice coverage.

Funding is certainly the biggest hurdle to initiating and continuing an OB/GYN hospitalist program. Looking at the direct net costs, this is not a profitable venture. However, judging by the rapid growth of this specialty and adoption by so many hospitals, the indirect benefits (improving care, lowering risk, and improving the labor and delivery environment with immediate availability of obstetric physicians), seem to outweigh this issue in the minds of the financial decision makers. Over time, especially if private physicians turn over the care for delivery of a number of their private patients, and that number continues to increase with time, the program can become solvent.

Training OB/GYN hospitalists presents a challenge for all of the various organizational structures. Currently, many programs defer hiring new residency graduates, because labor and delivery skills and judgment are perceived to be lacking in this group. Older, more experienced clinicians who are at least 5 years out of residency are often preferred. Regardless, the need for additional training to focus on this new subspecialty, especially the need for critical care skills, operative delivery skills, knowledge and expertise in fetal heart rate monitoring, and other areas specific to labor and delivery need to be honed for optimal performance of the OB/GYN hospitalists. OB/GYN hospitalist medicine may become a new subspecialty of obstetrics and gynecology and fellowship training and board certification will follow. There are currently at least 2 university-based fellowship training programs for OB/GYN hospitalists.[9,10]

Staffing is always a potential problem for this subspecialty. Because most programs will only need 1 OB/GYN hospitalist on duty at all times, about 4.5 full-time equivalent positions are needed to adequately staff a unit. There is often a mix of full- and part-time hospitalists, or 5 to 7 individuals covering the call schedule. But when one of these clinicians is out because of illness or another reason, finding a temporary replacement quickly is often difficult. Universities and staff model organizations have the most flexibility, and coverage may also be found temporarily in private hospitals from private physicians, regardless of the organizational model. Physician practice management companies have available pools of physicians for locum tenans. For more permanent replacements, there is generally less of a problem, because the ratio of applicants to position remains high at this time.

Private physician acceptance is primarily a problem in initiating and sustaining OB/GYN hospitalist programs. This problem is the greatest in hospital-run programs, but is similar when hospitals seek outside groups or physician management companies to run their programs. The problem is less of an issue in university programs, where acceptance will be greatest, by MFM groups seeking inpatient extenders and by large staff model health maintenance organizations. The exception to the latter is in staff model programs, where physician compensation may depend on billing success and some physicians need labor and delivery call rotations to earn their compensation. For private physicians, the concern is certainly understandable. However, assuming for example an average of 12 deliveries a month for an obstetrician, with an average compensation of say $1800 for total obstetric care. If the clinician turns over many of his or her night and weekend deliveries and even some during the day; if the physician gives up 5 deliveries that month to the OB/GYN hospitalist and pays the hospitalist $500 per delivery, the private physician only needs to take on 1 to 2 new obstetric patients per month to make up the difference. And because most OB/GYN groups take on new partners, often because of night and weekend call pressures (as opposed to increasing patient volume), using the OB/GYN hospitalist is a far more cost-effective venture than the cost of salary and benefits for a new associate. In addition, there is the added productivity of staying in the office and seeing scheduled patients instead of attending to patients in labor.

Patient satisfaction is often an expressed concern of OB/GYN hospitalist programs, especially in private practice settings. The private physician often thinks that their patients expect their own physician to be present for their delivery. But in reality, many patients are already delivered by other physicians who provide call coverage, many of whom the patient has not met before. In patient satisfaction surveys[3,11] we are aware of, patients seem at least as happy with the OB/GYN hospitalist managing their labor and doing their delivery as compared with private practice, and anecdotally have expressed being pleased with meeting the OB/GYN hospitalist early in their labor process, being reassured that someone who knows the details of their case is around and immediately available, and will often come in and answer questions as opposed to someone who just shows up at the last minute for the delivery, as may happen in a private practice model. In other practice models, like universities, staff model practices, or MFM practices (especially with transfer of care or maternal transports), this issue is nonexistent. Continuity of patient care is one of the real disadvantages of the hospitalist type of model. The potential for a "shift mentality" to creep into practice is always present, tempting the less diligent and dedicated to put off decisions or interventions to the next shift. In addition, the continuity of following a patient, particularly those with complications, through the postpartum period is often lost; but this is not uncommon in other types of practices, like staff models, universities with various faculty covering at night and on weekends, and even in private practice where the on-call physician who attends the delivery or performs the procedure often does not follow the patient throughout her hospital stay.

Malpractice coverage is an issue in evolution. If malpractice claims remain constant, and knowing most obstetric claims arise in labor and delivery as opposed to in the outpatient setting, the 4 or 5 OB/GYN hospitalists covering the unit of say 300 to 400 deliveries per month will likely be exposed to a much greater number of cases (although the OB/GYN hospitalist may not be the physician of record) and more likely to the most difficult and critical situations than if any of those individuals was just doing their own and partners deliveries of say 20 per month. Thus, the likelihood of exposure is potentially much greater for the hospitalist. To our knowledge, this pattern has not yet resulted a rate differential for OB/GYN hospitalists; nonetheless, the potential remains. In contrast, the most common allegations of negligence with neonatal encephalopathy developing shortly after birth relate to lack of immediate availability of the physician, delayed intervention, and problems with nurse–physician communication aggravated by the physician being off site. The OB/GYN hospitalist has the potential of greatly ameliorating these problems. The potential for OB/GYN hospitalists to reduce liability exposure and decrease adverse outcomes remains to be proven. In situations where the hospital employs the hospitalist and their insurance is covered by the hospital policy or the hospital is self-insured, the increased exposure of the hospitalist will be offset because the total number of cases remains the same. This same would apply to university programs and staff model practices. Thus, the concern over the increased exposure of the OB/GYN hospitalists is mainly for those types of hospitalist practices where the physicians are insured separately.

SUMMARY

This article has summarized the current state of business and organizational models of developing OB/GYN hospitalist practices and will be valuable for those programs currently starting a new program. We estimate that only about 10% to 20% of obstetric units with delivery volumes large enough to support an OB/GYN hospitalist program currently have one, although 1 survey estimated it to be as high as 38%.[12] There remains a large number of programs yet to consider and/or initiate this model and we hope the information provided in this article will help that process.

REFERENCES

1. Iriye BK, Huang WH, Condon J, et al. Implementation of a laborist program and evaluation of the effect upon cesarean delivery. Am J Obstet Gynecol 2013; 209(3):251.
2. Rosenstein M, Nijagal M, Nakagawa S, et al. The effect of expanded midwifery and hospitalist services on primary cesarean delivery rates. Abstract No. 8. Oral presentation at the Plenary Session of the 35th Annual Meeting of the Society for Maternal Fetal Medicine. San Diego, California, February 5–7, 2015.
3. Wachter RM, Goldman L. The hospitalist movement 5 years later. JAMA 2002; 287(4):487–94 Patient satisfaction.
4. OB Hospitalist group. Available at: www.obhg.com. Accessed June 15, 2015.
5. MedNax, Pediatrix/Obstetrix Medical Group. Available at: www.mednax.net. Accessed June 15, 2015.
6. Delphi of Team Health. Available at: www.teamhealth.com. Accessed June 15, 2015.
7. Quest Care. Available at: www.questcare.com. Accessed June 15, 2015.
8. D'Alton M, Bonanno C, Berkowitz R, et al. Putting the "M" back in MFM. Am J Obstet Gynecol 2013;208(6):442–8.
9. University of California Irvine Department of Obstetrics and Gynecology. Available at: https://recruit.ap.uci.edu/apply/JPF02466. Accessed June 15, 2015.
10. Winthrop University Department of Obstetrics and Gynecology. Available at: http://www.winthrop.org/departments/education/gme/rt-oag.cfm#hfp. Accessed June 15, 2015.
11. Srinivas SK, Jesus AO, Turzo E, et al. Patient satisfaction with the laborist model of care in a large urban hospital. Patient Prefer Adherence 2013;7:217–22.
12. Srinivas S, Lorch S. The laborist model of obstetric care: we need more evidence. Am J Obstet Gynecol 2012;207(1):30–5.

Obstetrics and Gynecology Hospitalist Fellowships

Anthony M. Vintzileos, MD

KEYWORDS

- Obstetrics and gynecology • Hospitalist • Fellowship • Patient safely
- Physician satisfaction

KEY POINTS

- The primary aim of OB/GYN hospitalist fellowships is to train physicians in a way that aligns their interests with those of the hospital with respect to patient care, teaching, and research.
- OB/GYN hospitalist fellowship programs will provide extra training and confidence for recent residency graduates who want to pursue a hospitalist career.
- OB/GYN hospitalist fellowship programs will support the increasing needs for OB/GYN hospitalists, improve patient care and safety, and increase physician satisfaction.

INTRODUCTION

The enormous proliferation of managed care over the past 3 decades has resulted in the need for judicious use of health care resources and cost reduction. This has led to several changes in practice patterns to maintain efficiency and patient safety. Under these circumstances and because most resources are spent in acute hospital settings, it is not surprising that physicians dedicated to hospital work have become key players in an effort to provide high-value health care. Acute hospital settings include emergency rooms, critical care units, postoperative units, and labor and delivery (L&D) suites. As a result, there have been an increasing number of physician hospitalists from many specialties and subspecialties, such as general internal medicine, pediatrics, critical care, surgery, neurology, and obstetrics and gynecology (OB/GYN).[1,2] A survey in 2011 showed that 13.3% of primary care physicians were hospitalists and that between 2009 and 2011 the percentage of hospital admissions for Medicare patients increased from 25.7% to 31.8%.[3]

Disclosure Statement: The author reports no conflicts of interest.
Department of Obstetrics and Gynecology, Winthrop University Hospital, 259 First Street, Mineola, NY 11501, USA
E-mail address: avintzileos@winthrop.org

Obstet Gynecol Clin N Am 42 (2015) 541–548
http://dx.doi.org/10.1016/j.ogc.2015.05.012
0889-8545/15/$ – see front matter

obgyn.theclinics.com

The term "hospitalist" was coined by Wachter and Goldman in mid 1990s in an article written for the University of California, San Francisco, resident's "newsletter" and a year later in an official article published in the *Journal of the American Medical Association*.[3,4] Hospitalists work and provide patient care in the hospital. Their role is to make sure that hospital protocols and guidelines are followed appropriately, to coordinate care, and to improve communication during transitioning of care, thus improving efficiency and patient safety. The challenges for hospitalists are to minimize the use of unnecessary tests and at the same time maintain or improve outcomes. A retrospective historical cohort study has shown that a system using full-time hospitalists may significantly decrease the hospital stay, readmission rate, and overall medical cost of care without any negative effect on patient satisfaction.[1,5,6]

The first publication regarding hospitalists in OB/GYN was by Weinstein,[7] who pointed out the need for "laborists" who would concentrate on managing patients in labor. The main reasons for laborists included a projected shortage of obstetricians who deliver infants due to increasing rates of burnout and the medical legal crisis. Additional speculated benefits included improved patient outcomes and physician satisfaction. Indeed, subsequent research showed that OB/GYN hospitalists and laborists have higher job satisfaction as compared with nonhospitalists.[8] However, large prospective comparative studies of specific maternal and neonatal outcomes with and without laborists are needed to understand the impact of the laborist model.[9]

In a 2010 committee opinion, the American College of Obstetricians and Gynecologists supported the model of care by OB/GYN hospitalists and opined that this model of care will most likely result in physician and patient satisfaction and at the same time will provide effective and safe patient care.[10] The document clarified the term "laborist" as being a physician whose primary responsibility is to manage patients in labor and with obstetric emergencies and "OB/GYN hospitalist" as being a physician whose responsibility is expanded to include emergent gynecologic care of hospitalized OB/GYN patients.

Although the needs for laborists and OB/GYN hospitalists is rapidly increasing,[11] their mean age in a 2010 survey was 48.8 years and the average number of years since their residency was 17.0 years.[8] As a result, it is likely that in the near future there may be a shrinking pool of available hospitalists, given the increasing demand and the fact that recent residency graduates very rarely are choosing to become hospitalists. Possible reasons why recent OB/GYN residency graduates do not choose a hospitalist career is because many of them chose to pursue Accreditation Council for Graduate Medical Education (ACGME)-approved OB/GYN fellowships or because they may not feel equipped or feel they have the necessary experience to manage rare complications. There is no question that the limits in resident work hours that have been imposed on training programs over the past decade must have had a negative effect on resident experience, because the length of training remained the same at 4 years. This lack of experience is mostly for rare obstetric and surgical emergencies. After consideration of all these issues, an OB/GYN hospitalist fellowship may provide a safe "bridge" for those who are interested in a hospitalist career, especially for recent OB/GYN resident graduates.

STEPS UNDERTAKEN TO CREATE THE FIRST OBSTETRICIAN/GYNECOLOGIST HOSPITALIST FELLOWSHIP

Since 2010, Winthrop University Hospital had established an OB/GYN Hospitalist Division within the Department of Obstetrics and Gynecology consisting of 2 senior and very experienced OB/GYN physicians. The challenge was to build the educational component for the hospitalist fellowship. The first step was to form a core group of interested physicians who believed in the need for an OB/GYN Hospitalist fellowship. This core physician group consisted of the following 8 members:

- Chairman with subspecialty of maternal-fetal medicine (MFM)
- The chief of obstetrics, who also carries the responsibility of quality/safety officer
- The OB/GYN residency director (subspecialty MFM)
- A senior gynecologist (trained in robotics and simulation)
- Two senior gynecologists (trained in robotics)
- Two senior general OB/GYN hospitalists

The second, and most challenging, step was to secure funding. Because Winthrop University Hospital was "over the cap" for residency slots, the idea of the fellowship, along with a business plan, was presented to the chief executive officer of the hospital. After securing the funding for the fellow's salary (at the postgraduate year 5 level), the rationale for creating the fellowship, as well as the goals and objectives of the fellowship program, were presented to the Winthrop Graduate Medical Education (GME) Committee for approval. In January of 2013, the GME committee of Winthrop University Hospital approved a 1-year OB/GYN hospitalist fellowship starting July 1, 2013. Between January and July 2013, the core group of physicians met several times to determine the goals and objectives of the fellowship program. During these deliberations, consultation was also sought from the academic committee of the Society of OB/GYN Hospitalists, because they were in the process of also developing core competencies for OB/GYN hospitalists. Recruitment efforts involved e-mailing OB/GYN residency program directors, as well as placement of ads in "OB/GYN News" and also in our 2 main journals (Obstetrics and Gynecology and American Journal of Obstetrics and Gynecology). The ads indicated that the candidate fellows should have completed an American Board of Obstetrics and Gynecology–approved OB/GYN residency program and also have a New York medical license or permit. We had 20 responses and conducted 4 interviews. Our first selected fellow was a June 2012 graduate from Jersey City Medical Center, who started the hospitalist fellowship on July 1, 2013, and successfully completed it on June 30, 2014.

LEARNING OBJECTIVES OF THE OBSTETRICIAN/GYNECOLOGIST HOSPITALIST FELLOWSHIP
General Learning Objectives

The goal of the OB/GYN hospitalist fellowship program curriculum at Winthrop University Hospital is to provide fellows with the experience, knowledge, and skills necessary to practice as OB/GYN hospitalists. The learning objectives are linked to the 6 ACGME competencies, including medical knowledge, patient care, professionalism, interpersonal and communication skills, practice-based learning, and improvement and systems-based practice. The expectation is that the program will provide the graduating fellow with all the necessary competences to work independently in the hospital environment. The entire training is provided at Winthrop University Hospital.

Specific Learning Objectives

Quality Improvement and Patient Safety is the guiding principle in the curriculum of the OB/GYN hospitalist fellow. The goal of the program is to ensure competence of the fellow graduate in managing the clinical problems of OB/GYN-hospitalized patients and in improving the performance of the hospital and its health care systems by

- Prompt and complete attention to all patient care needs, including diagnosis, treatment, and the performance of medical procedures under appropriate supervision;
- Use of quality and process improvement techniques;
- Collaboration, communication, and coordination with all residents, fellows, and attending physicians and health care personnel caring for hospitalized patients;
- Safe transitioning of patient care within the hospital, and from the hospital to the community;
- Efficient use of hospital and health care resources;
- Developing expertise in drills and simulation;
- Developing expertise in conducting systems-based morbidity and mortality reviews (practice-based learning and improvement);
- Developing the key qualities of teamwork, quality improvement, and leadership; and
- Conducting research and or developing tools to improve the perinatal and other OB/GYN patient care core measures as defined by national organizations such as National Quality Forum, Medicaid, and Medicare. **Box 1** lists the specific core measures that are the focus of the fellow's efforts toward research and quality improvement.

Clinical duties
Under the supervision of the hospitalist attending physician, the fellow has a variety of clinical duties, which are summarized in **Box 2**.

Educational duties
The educational duties of the fellow are summarized in **Box 3**.

FELLOWSHIP PROGRAM EVALUATION

The fellow is given verbal feedback on a daily basis. Official evaluations are completed every 3 months (electronically) by the core faculty members of the OB/GYN Hospitalist Division, as well as private attendings and faculty members who had the opportunity to work with the fellow. The fellow evaluation (Core Clinical Competence) committee

---

Box 1
Hospitalist fellow's core measures for research and quality improvement

- Elective deliveries at less than 39 weeks
- Cesarean deliveries in nulliparous patients with a term, singleton fetus in vertex position
- Antenatal steroids in preterm births at 24 to 32 weeks
- Health care–associated infections in hospitalized OB/GYN patients
- Exclusive breastfeeding during hospitalization
- Antibiotic prophylaxis within 1 hour before incision for OB/GYN surgeries
- Appropriate VTE prophylaxis
- Intrapartum antibiotics for GBS prophylaxis
- Readmissions of OB/GYN patients

Abbreviations: GBS, group B streptococcus; OB/GYM, obstetrics/gynecology; VTE, venous thromboembolism.

Box 2
List of clinical duties of the OB/GYN hospitalist fellow

- Sign out all triage patients and personally evaluate these patients, as needed
- Manage unexpected obstetric emergencies, such as an obstetric hemorrhage, prolapsed cord, shoulder dystocia, cesarean hysterectomies, and operative deliveries
- Be available to manage labor, not just attend deliveries
- Evaluate admitted patients, write an admitting note or history and physical examination and initial orders, and order all nonroutine laboratory and other tests
- Monitor patients' labor progress, complications, need for anesthesia, and need for amniotomy
- Work jointly with the patients' private physicians
- Decide and implement labor interventions (eg, oxytocin or amnioinfusion), review fetal monitor strips (especially when any abnormality or concern is noted by the nurse and any time any nonsurgical intervention is required), decide on the need for internal monitoring, and be present for emergent deliveries
- Assist on operative deliveries, twins, or other procedures
- Assist with neonatal resuscitation in unanticipated situations
- Evaluate and manage postpartum complications
- Check on hospitalized antepartum patients
- Provide ongoing nursing and physician education
- Be on-call for the general OB/GYN emergency room
- Perform emergent gynecologic surgery for cases such as ectopic pregnancies or incomplete abortion curettage
- Provide emergency room consultations and/or emergency surgical procedures for gynecologic patients
- Be responsible for unassigned inpatient gynecologic patients or referred gynecologic patients from private physicians
- Perform emergent OB/GYN ultrasounds
- Facilitate "Obstetric Safety" rounds on L&D daily
- Participate in TeamSTEPPS on L&D the third Friday of every month
- Facilitate gynecologic morning resident sign-out rounds
- Be available for in-house call 4 shifts a month

Abbreviations: L&D, labor and delivery; OB/GYN, obstetrics/gynecology; TeamSTEPPS, Team Strategies and Tools to Enhance Performance and Patient Safety.

---

meets every 3 months to discuss the fellow evaluations and progress. The following competences of the fellow are evaluated: patient care, clinical and surgical skills, medical knowledge, practice-based learning and improvement, interpersonal and communication skills, professionalism, systems-based practice, and teaching skills. The Core Clinical Competence Committee consists of the director of the hospitalist fellowship, the chief of quality for obstetrics, the OB/GYN residency program director or designee, and 1 to 2 private OB/GYN physicians who have worked closely with the fellow. The fellow evaluates the program every 3 months electronically and the day-to-day training program is modified accordingly so as to improve the fellow's

---

Box 3
Educational duties of the OB/GYN hospitalist fellow

- Supervise and teach OB/GYN residents and students
- Participate in all simulations and drills (the first 6 months the fellow will be taught and the last 6 months will be a teacher)
- Simulation center training with residents the second and fourth Fridays of each month
- Participate in using the laparoscopic trainer, Noelle birth simulator, and neonatal resuscitation simulation
- Participate in resident pig laboratory simulation training 4 Fridays in the first half of the year
- Perform 1 student lecture per student block
- Become NCC, NALS, BLS, ACLS certified
- Participate as a member and representative of the department in the following monthly committee meetings: OR Committee, Hospital-Wide Patient Safety Committee, Obstetric Quality Improvement Committee.

Abbreviations: ACLS, Advanced Cardiac Life Support; BLS, Basic Life Support; NALS, Neonatal Advanced Life Support; NCC, National Certification Corporation (for fetal heart rate monitoring); OB/GYN, obstetrics/gynecology; OR, operating room.

---

experience. **Table 1** provides a grid that shows our first weekly schedule, which was slightly modified in the subsequent year (2014–2015) to include outpatient follow-up of patients operated-on by the fellow because they had presented in the hospital with gynecologic surgical emergencies.

Table 1
Weekly fellow schedule (2013–2014)

Monday	Tuesday	Wednesday	Thursday	Friday	Saturday
6:30 AM Gyn sign-out rounds	7 AM–4 PM Block OR; Gyn Cases Backup to L&D	7 AM–12 PM L&D/ER consults	7 AM–4 PM L&D/ER consults	7 AM–12 PM Robotics 12 PM–4 PM L&D/ER consults	One 24-h in-house call per month
7 AM–4 PM L&D/ER consults	2nd Tues of each month QIAC meeting 1030–1130; OR Committee meeting 12 PM–1 PM	1st Wed each month 8 AM–9 AM Ob Improvement Committee meeting	—	Simulation Training as described above (**Box 3**); 10 AM–12 PM, 2 Fridays each month	—
—	3rd Tuesday of each month 12 PM–1 PM Hospital Patient Safety Committee meeting	12 PM–4 PM Research time	—	One 24-h in-house call per month	—

Abbreviations: ER, emergency room; Gyn, gynecology; L&D, labor and delivery; Ob, obstetrics; OR, operating room; QIAC, Quality Improvement Advisory Committee.

OUR FIRST HOSPITALIST FELLOW RESEARCH PROJECT

Our first hospitalist research project was presented during resident graduation day, along with the other resident research presentations, in June 2014. The fellow's research was a quality improvement project aiming to assess costs and obstetric outcomes in patients with unfavorable cervix requiring induction of labor. The comparison groups involved patients who had labor induction with 50 µg vaginal misoprostol versus those induced with 10 mg dinoprostone vaginal inserts. The study found that there were no differences in obstetric and neonatal outcomes. However, the misoprostol group had a statistically significant decreased time to active labor (median 8 vs 12 hours), time to delivery (median 11 vs 17 hours), and L&D stay (median 16 vs 24 hours). In addition, the use of misoprostol was associated with cost savings of approximately $440 per patient. This would translate to annual cost savings for the hospital of approximately $250,000 for a policy of using misoprostol as compared with dinoprostone. Here, it is important to emphasize that the hospitalist fellow's annual salary was (and continues to be) much less than $250,000. The results of this research project were presented to the Obstetric Improvement Committee and subsequently to the entire OB/GYN staff. A protocol using misoprostol was drafted, and residents, faculty, and private attending were encouraged to use misoprostol rather than dinoprostone for inductions of labor. Subsequent monthly monitoring revealed an increasing rate of misoprostol use for induction of labor from 30% to approximately 50%.

SUMMARY/DISCUSSION

We believe that the pool of OB/GYN hospitalists needs to be expanded in a drastic manner so as to accommodate the needs of the country. Creating OB/GYN hospitalist fellowships may very well address this need, although this is only speculative at this time and more data are needed. OB/GYN fellowship programs should provide extra training and confidence for recent resident graduates who want to pursue a hospitalist career. The primary aim of OB/GYN fellowships should be to train physicians in a way that aligns their interests with those of the hospital, with respect to patient care, teaching, and research. Research in the core measures should be a necessary component of the fellowship so as to provide long-term benefits for all stakeholders, including hospitals and patients.

REFERENCES

1. Wachter RM, Goldman L. The hospitalist movement 5 years later. JAMA 2002; 287:467–94.
2. Wachter RM. Reflections: the hospitalist movement a decade later. J Hosp Med 2006;1:248–52.
3. Welch PW, Stearns SC, Cuellar AE, et al. Use of hospitalists by Medicare beneficiaries; a national picture. Medicare Medicaid Res Rev 2014;4 [pii: mmrr2014.004.02.b01].
4. Wachter RM, Goldman L. The emerging role of "hospitalists" in the American health care system. N Engl J Med 1996;335:514–7.
5. Diamond HS, Goldberg E, Janosky JE. The effect of full-time faculty hospitalists on the efficiency of care at a community teaching hospital. Ann Intern Med 1998; 129:197–203.
6. Chaty B. Hospitalists: an efficient, new breed of inpatient caregivers. Healthc Financ Manage 1998;52:47–9.

7. Weinstein L. The laborist: a new focus of practice for the obstetrician. Am J Obstet Gynecol 2003;188:310–2.

8. Funk C, Anderson BL, Schulkin J, et al. Survey of obstetric and gynecologic hospitalists and laborists. Am J Obstet Gynecol 2010;203:177.e1–4.

9. Srinivas SK, Lorch SA. The laborist model of obstetrical care: we need more evidence. Am J Obstet Gynecol 2012;207:30–5.

10. ACOG committee opinion no. 459: the obstetric-gynecologic hospitalist. Washington, DC: American College of Obstetrics and Gynecology; 2010.

11. Olson R, Garite TJ, Fishman A, et al. Obstetrician/gynecologist hospitalists: can we improve safety and outcomes for patients and hospitals and improve lifestyle for physicians? Am J Obstet Gynecol 2012;207:81–6.

Index

Note: Page numbers of article titles are in **boldface** type.

A

Acute hypertensive crisis
   preeclampsia and
      maternal mortality related to
         OB-GYN hospitalists' in reducing, 470–472
Attending physician fatigue
   sleep deprivation–related, 499–502

B

Business and organizational models of OB-GYN hospitalist groups, **533–540**
   administration considerations related to, 535
   benefits of, 535
   described, 533–540
   differences in types of, 534–535
   funding of, 538
   malpractice coverage in, 539–540
   patient satisfaction as concern in, 539
   physician acceptance in, 538–539
   reasons for setting up, 534–535
   specific models, 537–538
   staffing in, 538

C

Cesarean delivery
   OB-GYN hospitalists in, 478–483
      neonatal outcomes related to, 482–483
      rates of delivery, 480–481
      in trial of labor following, 480–483. *See also* Trial of labor after cesarean delivery
        (TOLAC)
      vaginal birth following, 480–483

D

Delivery
   in emergent situations
      timeliness of
         OB-GYN hospitalists in, 489
Device-associated morbidity
   hospitalists' impact on, 435

Obstet Gynecol Clin N Am 42 (2015) 549–555
http://dx.doi.org/10.1016/S0889-8545(15)00069-8
0889-8545/15/$ – see front matter © 2015 Elsevier Inc. All rights reserved.

obgyn.theclinics.com

Moving?

Make sure your subscription moves with you!

To notify us of your new address, find your **Clinics Account Number** (located on your mailing label above your name), and contact customer service at:

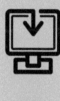

Email: journalscustomerservice-usa@elsevier.com

800-654-2452 (subscribers in the U.S. & Canada)
314-447-8871 (subscribers outside of the U.S. & Canada)

Fax number: 314-447-8029

Elsevier Health Sciences Division
Subscription Customer Service
3251 Riverport Lane
Maryland Heights, MO 63043

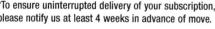
*To ensure uninterrupted delivery of your subscription, please notify us at least 4 weeks in advance of move.

ELSEVIER

Printed and bound by CPI Group (UK) Ltd, Croydon, CR0 4YY

03/10/2024

01040497-0013